LIGHT AEROBICS EXERCISES

For Seniors and the Lazy Man!

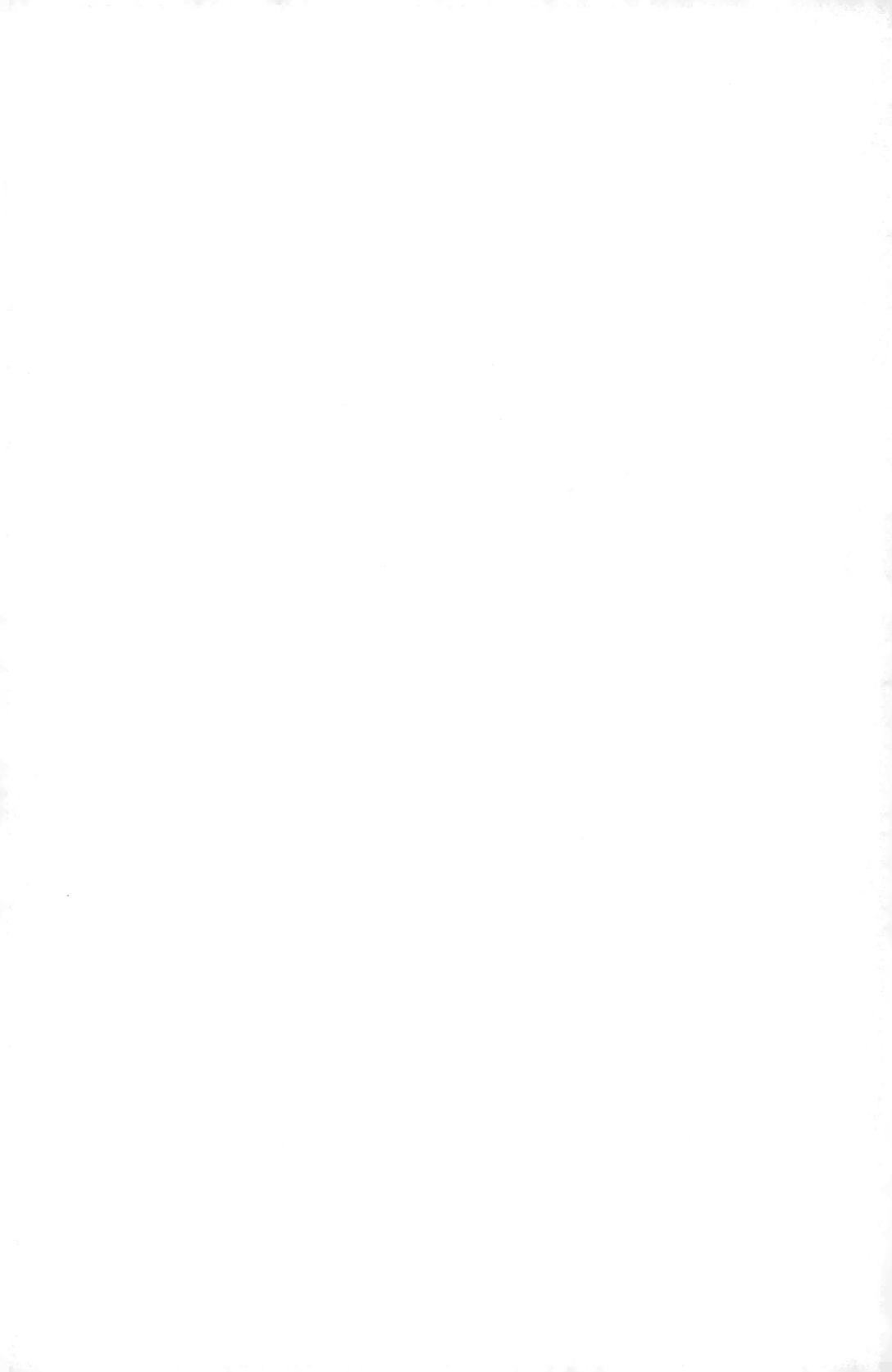

LIGHT AEROBICS EXERCISES

For Seniors and the Lazy Man!

Jaime E. Arcebuche

This book was printed in the United States of America.

(719) 3445025; Email: arcebuche@yahoo.com

To order additional copies of this book, contact:
Xlibris Corporation
1-888-795-4274
www.Xlibris.com
Orders@Xlibris.com
105100

If You Have But One Choice for An Exercise Program, This Is For you!
An Exclusive & Confidential Copy For

_____

LIGHT AEROBICS EXERCISES For Seniors and the Lazy Man!

(A Unique Blending of the Most Common Exercise Practices
in the Oriental And Occidental Hemispheres.)

CAUTION: To be performed only after proper consultations-With a physician-or qualified Instructor. Anyone wishing to avail of this program must agree and sign his/her consent to the provisions herein outlined and return this page to the author for his release and authority.

The exercise and health practices suggested in this pamphlet should not be construed to supplant or replace any on-going treatment or rehabilitation program for any individual; the author or his authorized Representatives to be held blameless and free from any damages, suits or torts from any or all forms should any harm or injury befall anyone not under their personal supervision or tutelage with corresponding compensations.

The entire exercise system suggested herein may be completed, with reasonable proficiency, within Sixty minutes. For starters, this may be performed every other day for a month, after which, a maintenance program of twice a week is suggested.

Done properly, your body should be able to restart its natural healing processes and hopefully restore you to health without the use of drugs, alcohol or other stimulants, save those prescribed by your physicians. Should you feel any discomfort or negative effects in your system while doing this regimen, immediately inform your doctor about it.

This Document or any parts thereof may not be reproduced, circulated or copied in any form without the expressed written consent of the Author.

RELEASE AUTHORIZED BY:

_____

(Printed Name)

_____

(Signature & Date)

CONFORME' & APPROVED BY:

_____

(Signature & Date)

_____

(Printed Name)

• •

To Potential Recipients of this manuscript:

Should you come across this copy or a portion of it, this is being circulated to you In Confidence and may not be redistributed, copied in any form or manner, in whole or in part, without the expressed written consent of the AUTHOR. Possession of this copy means that you have already signed the Title page which includes the Authority and Release of the Author, otherwise, you are obliged to return it in person or by post within a period of One week upon receipt or possession of the same. For Email or electronic transfers, should you decide not to pursue this program, kindly DELETE it from your files and Inform the Author by Email about it.

Should you wish to avail of the Benefits of this Exercise regimen, please contact or arrange the same with the Author or his duly Authorized Representatives.

We disclaim any responsibility for any harm, injury or damage of any kind should this Program be used without the Author's or his Representatives' written Authority, the same to be held blameless and free from any and all legal damages, suits, torts and any or all form of accusations arising from its unauthorized use or applications.

The subjects herein covered are suggestive and recommendatory only. It basically reflects upon the author's own experiences and opinions. We do not claim any medical expertise or assurances of cure or healing, the best authority being your own physicians.

Should you wish for any further clarification, do not hesitate to contact the Author. The foregoing Caveats are only meant to protect those who just desire to spread the benefits of this Program.

We thank you in advance for your kind interest and hopefully, your learned feedback to also help benefit others.

Very truly yours,

JAIME E. ARCEBUCHE

Table of Contents

MAP OF SOUTHEAST ASIAN REGION

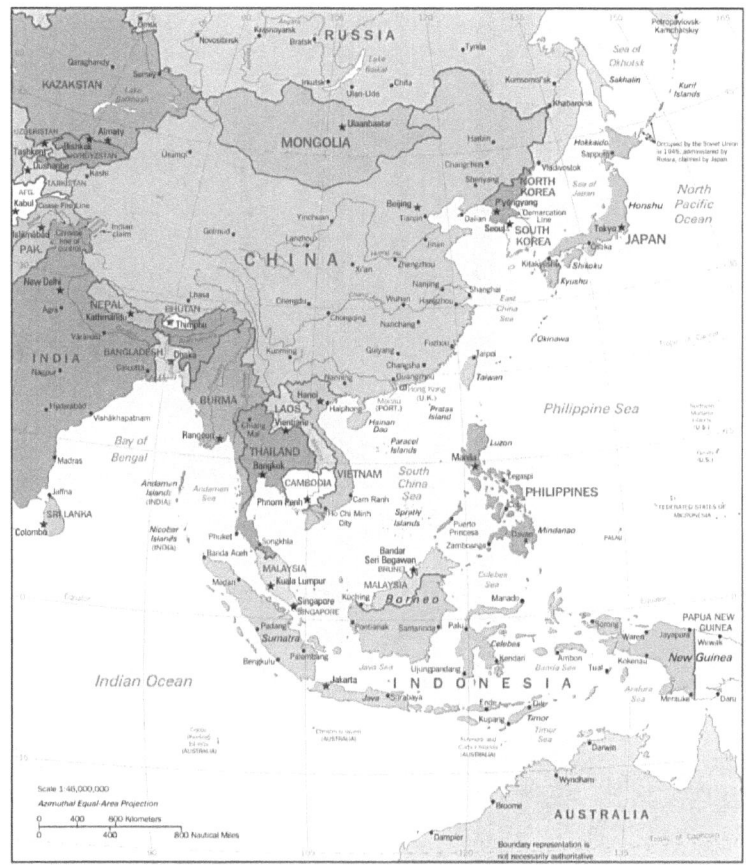

PHOTO TAKEN FROM AFE.ASIA.COLUMBIA.EDU

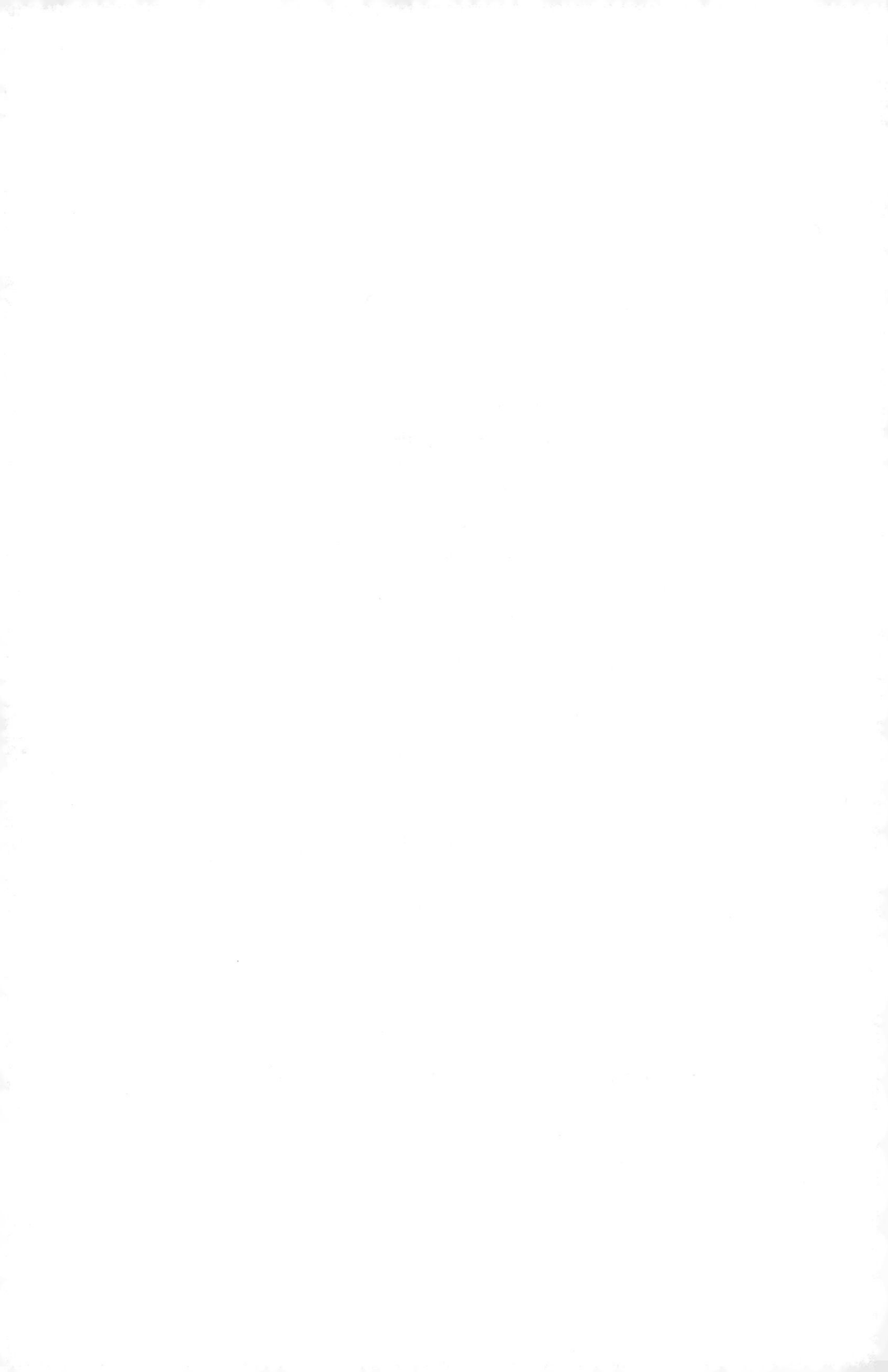

Dedication

TO ALL THE **SENIOR CITIZENS** OF THE WORLD,
WETHERSOEVER DESPERSED!
WE DON'T HAVE TO PROVE ANYTHING
TO ANYONE ANYMORE.
BIN DER, DON DAT!
THIS BOOK IS DEDICATED TO ALL OF YOU!

<u>CONFIDENTIAL CAVEAT FOR READERS OF</u>:

<u>IF YOU HAVE BUT ONE CHOICE FOR AN EXERCISE REGIMEN, THIS IS FOR YOU!</u>

This book is designed to integrate the most popular Aerobics-based exercises from the Oriental regimen and the Western-style systems, accomodate the complementary formats to establish a unique blend adoptable for busy workers, seniors and the lazy man!

The entire exercise system suggested herein may be completed, with reasonable proficiency, within Forty Five minutes or less. For starters, we recommend that it be performed every other day for at least a month, after which, a maintenance program of twice a week may suffice.

Done properly, your health permitting, your body should be able to restart and resume its natural healing capabilities that could hopefully restore back your regular vigor without the use of drugs (save those prescribed by your physician), alcohol, other stimulants and costly exercise equipment! It can performed in the privacy of your home, office, vehicle, in parks and public places whenever possible. Results could be tangible within weeks!

Should you feel any discomfort or experience any negative effects in your body while performing this exercise, immediately inform your physician about it.

The exercise and health practices suggested in this book should not be construed to supplant or replace any on-going treatment or rehabilitation programs prescribed by your doctor. Anyone who avails of this program is cautioned to consult with proper medical advice from competent health professionals. The author or his representatives is to be held blameless and free from any or all forms of legal or extra-legal suits or torts resulting from harm or injury that could befall to anyone not under their personal tutelage or supervision.

JAIME E. ARCEBUCHE
Author.

ACKNOWLEDGMENT

I wish to extend my gratitude to MS. LYNN SCHENTREUPP, formerly of the Arts Department of Hopkinsville High School, Hopkinsville, KY for the Line Art Drawings she kindly helped furnish my manuscript for the Full Body Exercise Regimen.

Ms. HYLAS (Holly) DOREY of Fountain City, Colorado, drew the segment of Finger Exercises (Mudras) included in this book as a personal favor.

I owe both Ms. Schentreupp and Ms. Dorey my eternal gratitude for their valued assistance.

The Indonesian art of TETADA KALIMASADA started me off in my search for alternative health practices in Southeast Asia, (Manila, Philippines), with the guiding principles of Grandmaster Pak Eddy Surohadi and his charming wife Dr. Ida Widyastuti Surohadi on the art of Self-Healing through proper exercise and deep breathing. They were effectively assisted by the Mother & son team of Cora Tinio and Jimmy Tinio, at their Makati Center.

The initial diagnosis of Dr. Lingling Uy, chief cardiologist of the University of the East's Ramon Magsaysay Memorial medical facilities in the Philippines and past President of the Philippine Cardiologists Association, were a shocking revelation for me.

I'm equally indebted to Dr. Kenneth H. Copper, former Chief medical officer of the US Air Force's Astronaut Training Program, considered as the "Father of Aerobics Exercise". I quoted exerpts from his book, "THE AEROBICS PROGRAM FOR TOTAL WELL-BEING". Ditto for Dr.Harvey B.Simon, author of "The No-Sweat Exercise Plan: Lose Weight, Get Healthy and Live Longer".

On the segment called "Suggested Food and Nutrition Reminders", I also quoted that portion on "Nutrition", from a publication of the

National Heart, Lung and Blood Institute (NHLBI) in an article authored in Heart Health by Beth Howard. On the subject about COFFEE-3 tricks to make it Super-Healthy, I am indebted to Mr.Mike Geary, author of "The Truth About Six-Pack Abs.".

The Map of the Asean Region was originally printed by the Columbian. edu and the ASEAN Secretariat.

Ms. Emma Price of the Sales Department of Xlibris was pivotal in my decision to have this book finally published when she outlined the most beneficial package for me. Ms. Goldie Dawson, Author's Representative was really patient with my incessant corrections and changes, even calling me up to discuss my latest editing efforts. Ms. Jill Suazo of Marketing Department was in the forefront of directing the Sales and Promotion efforts for this book. Mr. Jack Lora and Mr. Leo Bandala of the Corrections Department were competent in preparing the ever-changing texts, while Rhester Suelto & Bryan Villarin made an excellent rendition of the Front and Back Cover Designs. This competent team is under the able leadership of Ms. Vanessa Eugenio, Supervisor of the Customer Services Department. Kudos to all of them!

To all other pioneers of Aerobics exercise, health and nutrition, I extend my gratitude to them for helping me better understand the proper functions of the human body.

Finally, I was inspired to write about my readings, research and personal experiences by all the Senior Citizens of the world who are lazybones like me when it comes to the issue of a sustained exercise regimen, proper diet and healthful living. After well over eleven years, this book is now a reality!
To the lazy men and women of the world, I salute you!

JAIME E. ARCEBUCHE
Author

Foreword

Confident that I am about to write the next exercise book bestseller, I showed the manuscript to a friend from Cape Cod, Massachusetts which elicited this reaction, "Aha, another exercise manual. We seems to be getting more of it these days!". Out of curiosity, he took a second look. "Hmmm, says here it's for seniors and the lazy man! You pulling my leg? How can you do exercise if you're lazy?"

"Well, "I said excitedly, "just read on, it worked for me." Out of consideration, he give it a second look and scanned the first few pages, then commented, "My friend, there seems to be nothing new in this book. I'm from North America and its in here where many exercise regimen are learned. In fact, advances in health and medical science are made in these parts and all these new-fangled alien practices are to me, just that—foreign and mysterious!"

"You're absolutely right on both counts" I conceded. "In fact, I happen to agree wholeheartedly with you and have advocated most of these exercises practices in this book. They are all commendable." Then, I went on. "You must not debunk the merits of the exercise practices from other parts of the world, just because you are not familiar with them. I happened to have studied and practiced a few of these disciplines and found them to have unique benefits to the human body and, in fact could be complementary with Western-style exercise regimen." He leafed through the pages.

"What if" I pushed on, "a regimen can be devised where the more popular programs in both hemispheres can be combined to blend the two disciplines into one compleat system that is easy and practical, reducing the need to purchase costly exercise equipment, medicines, training or consultations? What if a simple program can be performed at home, at work, in school, in the park, in your car and even in your bed, for say, a couple of hours a week? Will this not be a win-win situation?" Having whetted his interest, I really poured it on. "And furthermore, within ninety days or less, you will sense an improvement in your metabolism, such that you could be taking fewer visits to your doctors or hospital, recover your regular sleeping patterns. Minor ailments like colds and headaches cured in shorter periods, help control stress and weight, prevent the onset of serious diseases, an improved mental attitude, faster grasp of ideas, etc. and get this, help alleviate sexual dysfunction?" He knitted his brows and said, "You pulling my leg?"

I smiled back and said, "Let me tell you a story, my friend."

Chapter I

MY STORY

With my background, I should be one of the last persons to trumpet on the merits of exercise and proper diet. My training was in the field of mechanical engineering and was physically active during my younger years. In later life however, I developed the love for unhealthy foods, lived a sedentary life, slept late and was a regular coach potato! I had no regular or even sporadic health regimen to speak of for admittedly, in this field I was a lazy man.

I hail from a central point in Southeast Asia, specifically from the Philippines—a marvelous archipelago of some seven thousand islands spread over an area less than the size of the state of Arizona. Its strategic location made it the convergence for early commerce and trade for neighboring nations among the Pacific-rim countries consisting of the Indo-Malayan peninsula and nations abutting the China Sea. Military leaders considered the country as the choke point of the Pacific hence, early maritime powers coveted it. Since its discovery by world-navigator Ferdinand Magellan and his Malayan guide, Enrique de Malacca on March 16, 1521, it became the territory of Spain for the next three hundred and fifty years. After the Spanish-American war, the Philippines, together with Cuba, Puerto Rico and Guam, were ceded by Spain to the United States for $20 million at the Treaty of Paris, becoming an American colony in 1898 until granted her independence on July 4, 1946.

In retrospect, while its geographical location is in Southeast Asia, its prevailing culture was predominantly Hispanic and for the last century, American-oriented. During all these period, its inhabitants continued to enjoy trade and immigration from neighboring countries thus, a hodge-podge of various influences pervaded among its people. The laid-back traits of the Christian Spaniards, with their siestas and fiestas; the mercantile and entrepreneurial Chinese traders; the reclusiveness of the Muslim inhabitants at its Southern backdoor and in later years, the pervasive presence of American servicemen assigned at the Subic Bay naval base in Olongapo City and the Clark air Force Base in adjacent Pampanga province, made the country a melting pot for various cultures.

Thus, in many metropolitan areas today, you will see the ubiquitous shopping centers with fast-food chains like Mcdonalds, KFCs, Wendys, Burger Kings, Chinese noodles centers, Japanese, Indian, Indonesian, Korean, Indian and Arabic cuisines in profusion, in competition beside native delicacies or combinations of them. In this tropical setting, you throw in a balmy climate, a year-round sunshine, sandy beaches all over and a hodgepodge of some eighty major local dialects among over 100 million inhabitants and you will see an interesting cultural variety in practice and in real time!

This diversity helped influence the growth of a people—its culture, language, traditions, tastes and yes, even medicine and exercise preferences. It was in this kind of cultural blend that somehow spawned my interest to read and got to know more about people from nearby and distant lands. Through the printed word, I was able to roam the various wonders of the world and its people. Through pictures and the medium of radio and television, I paid them more intimate visits. From the comfort of my easy chair, I was able to follow the many discoveries in science and technology. I was amazed at the strides made by medicine to help ease human suffering and prolong life. I also learned the importance of proper diet, regular exercise, proper life—style and the role of genetic heredity in personal wellness. All these, I followed keenly in my own sedentary way, even as I continued to watch television fueled by thick burgers, colas, French fries, noodles, pork-cracklings, and before retiring at night, my usual cup of sweetened caffeinated coffee! In due time, I began to experience the onset of debility. In my late fifties, I started to feel morose, shying away from social activities as my sex drive started to wane. Breathing became more labored, even when walking short distances and climbing up the stairs a few stories high. I stopped doing much productive work, didn't care much about making money and utterly felt miserable. As a stopgap concession to my physical deterioration, I had to quit on alcohol and smoking—cold turkey!

To compensate for it, I went on an eating binge—devouring more fast foods, colas, and frequent snacks and learned to love being a couch potato! Sounds familiar? Due to observed irregularity in my heartbeats, I paid a long-delayed visit with my heart physician, Dr., Lingling Uy, Chief Cardiologist of the University of the East's Ramon Magsaysay Memorial Medical center and a past president of the Philippines Cardiologists Association. When placed on a supervised treadmill routine, the test revealed a very sick heart. I was routinely informed that I needed a heart/lung bypass or worse, even a heart transplant operation! This woke me up real fast! I actually realized that I belong to family with an interesting heart history! (My late father, Gaudencio "Ading" Arcebuche died at the age of forty nine (49), while my younger brother, Henry Arcebuche kicked the bucket at age 45! He was also a picture of health and never suffered a stroke before. Presently, my younger sister, Dolores "Baby" de la Cruz was starting to experience heart issues too.

Even her active husband, William de la Cruz, got into the spirit of things and recently passed away at 68—from, you guess it, heart attack!) My youngest Sister, Nida A. Ocampo, younger brothers, Danilo Arcebuche and Alfredo (Boyet) have their own ailments but surpringsingly, didn't concerned heart issues.

Chapter II

UNRAVELING BAD NEWS!

News travel fast. My close personal friend, Abelardo L.Cruz, President of ALC Productions and her executive officer, Anna Magcalas, were then occupied with their weekly TV episodes entitled "Out Of Town", when they heard of my physician's diagnosis. Both immediately pounced on me to take this situation seriously, if I intend to join my children in the United States. Sensing of my relaxed attitude, Abel (codenamed: "Guerilla") immediately passed on the info to Engr.Jimmy P.Gilbuela (codenamed "Cactus"), our group's uncontested boogie rug-cutter and Chando P.Morallos (codenamed ("Ali") the unofficial Trini Lopez Version in the Philippines and writer with the Manila Daily Bulletin. Both paid me an immediate visits to inquire about steps I have taken about my heart issues. Unknowingly, my family driver, Esteban "Egoy" Castillo, Jr. confirmed my condition to them.

Bad news travels faster. For my apparent inaction, the reaction was immediate! My Masonic fraternity brother, Ill. Modesto D.Gonzales, 33rd, IGH promised to defeat me in all of our Scrabble Games with mutual friend, Val "Boy" Villavicencio; Ill. Bro. Ruben A. Azarcon, Sr., 33rd, IGH, a dentist, threatened to henceforth charge me for all dental services rendered if I don't shape up; while his son, Ill. Roy Azarcon, 33rd, IGH and wife Olga M. Azarcon echoed the same sentiments; Ill. Conrado "Rading" V.Sanga, 33rd IGH & lovely wife, Sis. Naty Sanga, were very much supportive, told me "We're always around and you can depend upon our help, should you need it". Ill. Reynaldo V. Paz 33rd IGH a Captain Pilot with the Philippines Air Lines, and his lovely wife, Sister Baby Labao Paz, pledged to drop me off at 10,000 feet without a parachute, while Bro. Gigi Ancajas, a bigwig in the Supreme Council.Order of DeMolay and connected with the Philippine Long Distance Telephone Company (PLDT), promised to yank my telephone off. These were meant to be serious threats should I pursue my present distant attitude about my ailment. Meanwhile, WB Felix Misa Bautista, PM, took me aside and whispered into my ear, "Bro, don't take them seriously. Let's go to my friend's place in Caloocan City's meat market who will prepare for us delicious meat finger foods with San Miguel Beer to go with it" and then silently sneaked me out from the madding crowd.

In the meantime, news started filtering into the higher echelons of Free-masonry. Now, past Grandmasters entered the act. MW. Raymundo N. Beltran, PGM and his wife, Sis. Luwalhati Beltran; MW Jose "Joe" R. Guerrero, PGM and spouse Sis. Aurora (Baby) P.Guerrero and MW Juan "Johnny" C. Nabong,Jr. PGM & Sis. Zeny Nabong, all heard it too, made inquiries and offered their assistance. So did a close friend and brother, VW Carlos "Charlie" R. de Castro, a well-known lawyer, rushed in to also asked how he could be of help! Even Noble Joe Rosales, an active Shriner from Hawaii, pitched in to offered assistance while friend and fraternity brother, Moly Ramajo & his wife, Eva Jane Ramajo, from far away Toronto, Canada, called me up (long distance) to confirm it and offered their assistance too.

When I visited my hometown in Catarman, Northern Samar, I was meet at the airport by Bro. Vicente Ortiz, 32nd and a Past Master of Northern Samar Masonic Lodge No. 211, who immediately asked me if the rumors were true. When I confirmed it, he picked up his wallet and inquired how much could I use. From the side, I espied my Compadre, Arthur "Baby" Uy, a respected local businessman in the company of my boyhood friend and neighbor, Engr. Francisco "Nonoy" Ladiao, who both signaled me with their fingers to join them. They similarly inquired about the news and having watched Bro.Vic Ortiz taking his wallet out, also had theirs on their hands. Both offered their financial assistance on—the—spot. "Baby Uy said, "this will just be the initial amount and if I sell my (coconut) Copra in Manila, you can have some more". I was of course grateful for their concerns, but I held my hand up and said "whoa!!!!! Hold your horses. Its as if I'm going under the knife soon. I havn't even secured a second opinion about it. At the moment, I feel just fine and hearty. Why don't we go fishing and afterwards drink glassfuls of Tuba, (a popular wine-like, sweet-tasting fresh extracts from budding coconut flowers.) They readily agreed, we went fishing and had a nice time!

(I made mention of these people who, unbidden came to me to offer assistance, for my readers of this exercise book to be aware that despite serious setbacks in our personal lives, there are always well-meaning friends and relatives who can be counted upon in dire situations.) I had no choice but to take my health issues seriously.

Later on, as my contemporaries started buying the farm, I took a second hard look at my lifestyle. Now, at the threshold of that human elite group called a senior citizen, I decided it was time for me to search and embrace other possibly less expensive and non-invasive health alternatives. With my condition, my body needed one major repair job. My other alternative was to delay treatment and to worry. Boy, did I worry!

It seemed that my health, my resolve and my finances, started to decline in exponential progression. Treading heretofore forbidden waters for me, I started to read more on health matters and watch allied subjects on television. Providentially, certain Far Eastern disciplines like Yoga, Tai-I chi, Qigong, Pranic healing. Acupuncture and some other aerobics exercises appeared to be having a resurgence among senior citizens like me.

As I've earlier pointed out, the Philippines is situated astride the geographical hub in Southeast Asia where the cacophony of cultural influences extend not only to language, culture, cuisine and religion, but even to the health and exercise preferences. With so many selections to choose from, the confusing array of options can be bewildering.

Now, here's when being a couch potato paid off! While watching a variety show on television one afternoon, I chanced upon a program that featured a group of senior citizens doing light aerobic exercises. While they appeared to be lithe, healthy and young looking, I just chalked it off to the effects of doing regular exercises regimen. Basically, nothing was new in there. What did caught my attention however, was a demonstration of what they termed as bio-energy, a latent force within the human body. When developed, they were able to demonstrate how it could manifest itself in some ways. One interesting example was dropping a brittle incandescent bulb to the cement floor. Normally, this fragile item will shatter when dropped, which it did. When another electric bulb was "coated" with the so-called bio-energy and dropped from shoulder level, the bulb just bounced off the cement floor, still intact!

Another demonstration featured a three-layer page of a daily newspaper that was spread on the floor and again, "coated" with bio-energy. A lady member was made to stand at the center while four others held on to the four corners of the paper. They slowly lifted it—and the lady atop the paper some two feet above the floor level and it held, without tearing apart. A more fantastic sidebar was shown when two cement bricks were place on its sides and a 20-watt fluorescent bulb suspended between the blocks. Again, it was "coated" with bio-energy and a 160-lbs. member was made to stand atop the center of the bulb. Miraculously, it held him up without breaking! Fantastic! I had to find this group.

Eventually, I located them doing bio-energy exercises on the fifth floor of a building without an elevator. This was my introduction to the Indonesian-style of bio-energy exercises called TETADA KALIMASADA! It appeared to consist of some light stretching maneuvers for the extremities, in conjunction with a form of breathing regimen. I signed in more for curiosity than an innate desire for exercise. After a couple of months, my metabolism seem to gradually improve. Continuing on with my program, I began to feel less subject to stress. My disposition started to get better, being less irritable and short-tempered. It seemed to me that more superior ideas and business concepts flew easily from my mind. Minor ailments seemed to heal faster. In time, I was able to walk twice the distance without the feeling of constrictions in my heart, climbed a few more stories higher, felt a bit more spry, and controlled my weight levels. More surprisingly, my sex drive gradually returned. Imagine, all these benefits without resorting to doctor's visits, drugs or pills? Wow!

A CLEAN BILL OF HEALTH

As a corollary benefit, I was able to harness my bio-energy potential and learned to perform the incandescent and fluorescent bulbs, as well as the newspaper lifting tricks! What was more amazing was just after six months from the time I embraced this exercise regimen, I went in for a more extensive physical examination. This was critical as the clinic, St. Luke's Medical Center, was retained by the United States Embassy in Manila to exclusively screen the health issues of visa applicants. To my surprise, their doctors pronounced me in great physical shape-a six-month wonder—boy! I could now look forward to attending my son's (Michael) wedding with Ms.Lourdes Flores in Toronto, Canada!

A more compelling reason was that, I now could accompany my granddaughter, N'cole Arcebuche, the three-year old charmer of my youngest son, Vincent Charles, a member of the United States Army and his wife, Gina C. Arcebuche. Undeniably, the family was ecstatic! I thanked my lucky stars for having stumbled upon a fantastic exercise regimen at the time when I was in desperate need for it! This was serendipity in real time!

I decided to take a closer look at other Oriental-based exercise programs and compared them with western-based ones. I noted a good many compatible findings in both disciplines. Western medicine is more empirical while the one from the Orient appeared to have some mystical and folklore components. I also discovered that both practices however, have their inherent strengths. Let's have a closer look at their common properties.

AEROBICS EXERCISES.

This refers to sustained activities that require the presence of large volume of oxygen in the circulatory system for prolonged periods, like pumping weights and short sprints. We are now aware that oxygen is the basic food component ingested for sustenance by our cells. Its longer presence in our body enables an improved time frame for our cells to avail itself of this food source. When doing *Aerobics*, muscular movements are performed while oxygen-laden air is entrapped under pressure within our *circulatory system*, poised to feed even inert or weakened cells and organs for their revitalization. This new paradigm of programmed breathing and the presence of high oxygen levels while doing exercises (in the West), was one obvious practice already routinely done and well-known from among the practitioners in the Orient. When regularly and properly performed at least 2-3 times a week, it can help further improve your metabolism by providing a faster exit venue for the system's wastes and toxic elements in the form of increased sweating, urination, stool movement and expulsion of dyspeptic gases (farting/burping).

This mode of doing exercise with dynamic breathing appears to be one effective way to heal and reactivate weakened cells and organs, which left unchecked, could result to weakness and debility. Prolonged presence of body wastes and toxins can eventually, be manifested in the form of ailments that doctors detects and treat—meaning pills, injections, ointments, massages, MRIs, X-rays, referrals, herbal cures, diets, esoteric exercise modules, more hospital visits and referrals and at times (horrors!) operations. It is said by certain writers that some of the treatments addressed the effects, rather than the causes, which, in many situations, may be traced to oxygen starvation! Now, ever wondered why the seemingly mystical practices of Tai-I-chi, Yoga, Kung Fu, Tetada Kalimasada, Reike, etc. have their obvious curative effects?

Many gurus in the medical field attest to the validity of exercise. My efforts to reconcile and complement these disparate systems led me to one proponent, noted author Dr. Kenneth H. Copper, former Chief medical officer of the United States Air force Astronaut's Training Program, also considered as the 'father' of Aerobics Exercise. In his book, "The Aerobics Program for Total Well-Being", he posited that "for me, the quest for total well-being began with the discovery of the amazing wonders of aerobic exercise—that is, endurance exercise which takes place over a relatively long period and depends on establishing a balance between the intake and expenditure of oxygen." He also pointed out that *Anaerobic* exercise (that is, without the prolonged presence of oxygen for short bursts) are performed, like a 100-meter sprint.

One other savant, Dr. Harvey B. Simon, author of "The No Sweat Exercise Plan: Lose Weight, Get Healthy and Live Longer" suggests a daily exercise program of 30 minutes.

Professional athletes learned to improve their endurance and performance levels by regular workouts, which helps them, sustain prolonged and increased oxygen levels in their system. Ditto for those in the military. Physical activity, coupled with proper diet and a healthy life-style can help ward off ailments too. Conversely, those of us who are not inclined to a regular regimen of exercise, proper diet and less healthy life styles, may be prone to certain ailments, most specially among seniors and the lazy man! But don't despair. Lazy men and women of the world, unite!

My research and personal experience helped me recover a portion of my earlier health levels with minimum access or consultations with physicians, nor the ingestion of prescription medicines, saved for a few routine ailments. In contrast, I witnessed the need of some friends and acquaintances for more trips to doctors and hospitals for a variety of benign or acute ailments, some even requiring operations. While this did not register with me early on, eventually it dawned upon me that I must be doing something right. With proper exercise, better ideas comes easily to mind. I've even became an autodidact. To learn more about the circumstances of my personal exercise program, I decided to skip my exercise regimen altogether for prolonged periods—sort of making my own body the object of an experimental study. My suspicions were then confirmed when there were corresponding recurrences of previous ailments and a general weakening of my systems against common ailments. Colds or headaches occurred with more frequency, requiring longer healing periods. My regular diet of gout, heartburn, backache and hyper-acidity ailments made their unwelcome presence known more often, despite my careful diet and healthier life style practices. Upon resuming my exercise regimen, the same ailments healed faster and the feeling of general well being, returned.

In making these observations, I cannot assert authoritative claims for its empirical accuracy, as I am not a trained medical practitioner. I can just make however, a testimonial for the positive results the program has given me and those of my friends who adhered to similar types of disciplines. You need not be an engineer or a certified mechanic to know that the preventive maintenance program you are doing for your own vehicle make it function with better efficiency and reliability. It is natural for people to share perceived situations and experiences with others, more especially when helping alleviate certain pains and ailments. Conditions and other factors vary, hence it would always be advisable for those who may wish to consider this exercise discipline to consult their physicians before, during and periodically thereafter.

Chapter III

THE DYNAMICS OF BREATHING.

Much of the observations I gleaned from my readings, the health-related television programs I watched and my varied exercise regimen, made me discern the common features fundamental to the art or science of healing. One of these I observed consists of the breathing techniques (that Dr. Kenneth Cooper defined as "establishing a balance between the intake and expenditure of oxygen" being performed while doing certain forms of exercise or even when at rest.

Breathing is fundamental to life. To stop breathing is to die. We ingest oxygen through breathing. Mr. M. R. de Haan of the DAILY BREAD MINISTRY observed that "adult lungs could hold some 5 liters of air, those of children, 3 liters. More often, you do not totally fill up or empty your lungs each time you breathe. Sitting at ease, your intake can be less than 500 cubic centimeters of air. When an adult takes a sprint, he breathes in about 90 liters a minutes, 15 times more than when relaxed. The same adult breathes in an average of 15,000 liters of fresh air everyday—about the volume contained in a boy's room, breathing some 23,000 times in 24 hours. This body fuel (oxygen) is required to power your heartbeat of 103,680 times in that period, circulating blood every 23 seconds, traveling some 43 million miles within your circulatory system while inhaling 438 cubic feet of air. In that same period, (of 24 hours), you digest 3 ½ lbs. of food, drink half a gallon of assorted liquids, evaporate two pounds of perspiration water, create 98.6 degrees of heat and generate some 450 tons of energy. You use 750 muscles, your hair grows 1/100 of an inch, and you will use 76 million brain cells!" This is the miracle of your body which we often take for granted. Systems failure are manifested in the form of ailments. It is our bounden duty to learn more about our body and how we can help it.

OXYGEN is the foundation of life. Our cells and organs feed upon it for sustenance to perform its assigned functions. When restricted of oxygen, a well-coordinated system is impaired, deteriorates and fail. Its temporary absence can cause ailments. Prolonged oxygen deprivation can lead to permanent debility or even death! How important is oxygen? Let's take a comparison. When you are deprived of food, you may live for as long as a few weeks; without water, maybe a few days—but, devoid of oxygen, less than an hour!

It becomes relevant to review at this point that *Aerobics* is the term used for exercise premised on the presence of oxygen in the respiratory system during bursts of activity. *Anaerobic* refers to the absence of oxygen. Elsewhere in this manuscript, I will recommend a more detailed style of breathing. This must be learned and mastered, because it is the superstructure upon which the entire regimen is firmly anchored upon. It basically consists of inhaling air slowly, pressing it downwards and storing it at the bottom of your lungs for a prolonged period, while doing bursts of activity for your *aerobics* exercises. Then, exhale air a bit longer, slowly.

Under these conditions (of holding your breath), even the extreme terminals of your *Respiratory System* can be reached by oxygen. The cells present along the small blood vessels and *alveoli*, when forced-feed through the simple act of pressing the air downwards & holding it at the bottom of your lungs (HDP) gives them a chance of better access to food (oxygen) that helps some inert cells and organs to recover or regenerate. Healthy cells leads to more vibrant organs that can readily perform its assigned functions with greater vitality. So, let's pull it for Oxygen!

COMPOSITION OF AIR.

The most abundant elements in the air is *Nitrogen* which comprises 78.048% in volume. Next is *Oxygen*, comprising 20.94%, *Argon* at 0.934%, *Carbon Dioxide* at 0.033%. Other *trace elements* comprising less than 20 parts per million include Neon, Helium, Krypton, Sulfur Dioxide, Methane, Hydrogen, Nitrous Oxide, Xenon, Ozone, Nitrogen Dioxide, Iodine, Carbon Monoxide and Ammonia.

HOW OXYGEN ENTERS THE BLOOD.

From among those elements in the air, our focus is on Oxygen, which when inhaled passes through our *Respiratory System*. It enters through the nose where it is warmed and filtered), the Pharynx, Trachea, Bronchi Tubes and the Lungs. Air can also be breathed through the mouth, via the larynx and on to the Trachea and lungs.

Within the lungs are the *Pleural membrane* and the *pleural cavity* where the real function of oxygen becomes beneficial to the body. Here, oxygen-laden air passes through the *Bronchial Tubes* which narrows down to the *Alveoli* consisting of a network of thin-walled membranes of small blood vessels called *Capillaries* where an exchange permits the cells in the blood a momentary contact with the air, releasing *Carbon dioxide* collected as wastes from the body, while taking in a fresh supply of oxygen which is food of the cells for distribution by the *Circulatory System* to the various organs of the human body.

EXPULSION OF BODY WASTES.

Deoxygenated blood from the heart is carried by cells through the plasma and again makes contact with the *Alveolus* where the exchange of Oxygen and Carbon Dioxide are made. The mechanics of breathing in and out is called *Ventilation*. Inhaling causes the chest muscles to contract, pulling and lifting the ribs outward. The *Diaphragm* then moves downward, enlarging the chest cavity to accept more air. A reverse process is made when air is exhaled or breathed out.

This process is being illustrated to give the reader a general profile on the powerful role that oxygen plays in our life. This in turn will help us appreciate the need for adhering seriously to the recommended *Breathing Dynamics* we are about to discuss that will be the basis of our Aerobics Exercise Program for the ailing, the busy workers, seniors and the lazy man!

THE *ARCEBUCHE-STYLE* OF AEROBICS AND DYNAMIC BREATHING TECHNIQUES.

All throughout this regimen, I have emphasized the use of my techniques of Breathing Dynamics as a pre-condition to our Aerobics and Bio-energy exercises. Perhaps, it would be more illustrative if I can share with you, the manner in which this type of technique (has) affected me. I believe that in due time, when the reader has already mastered the *system* as I had, it may have identical positive effects on them. In my particular situation, developing and mastering it did not come overnight but over a period of years of research, of discovery and of practice! In fact, it was just in the past year that I have managed to link it all together when *I* actually *felt* the instantaneous and beneficial effects of proper breathing. Now, I can share the techniques with you in this more detailed and systematic way. When breathing is integrated into the exercise system, this is what distinguishes the *Arcebuche-Style* of Light Aerobics & Systems' Restoration Routines from other similar formats. Having synthesized a variety of breathing styles and techniques through the years, I have now narrowed it down to the most effective manner in which my bodily systems have reacted favorably with. To revisit the technique, two main reasons were advanced at the onset of this regimen.

PREPARATORY LEVEL AND RATIONALE—When you embark upon any form of exercise, or even just going about your daily activities, your body performs certain tasks that require the coordination and efficient performance of its various organs and delivery functions. This series of automated activities is one fantastic miracle that performs unbidden within the confines of your body. To know and understand them will make you better appreciate the wonders of this new exercise paradigm.

As you perform your exercise, the *Respiratory System* ingests oxygen-laden air to replenish fuel to the cells carried in your bloodstream. Your *Lymphatic System* helps pick up unwanted debris and carbon dioxide, which are then exhaled out into the air. *The Circulatory or Cardiovascular system* distributes filters and cleanses the blood of wastes and other harmful elements before it completes back its circuit to feed the needed fuel to your cells and organs. Your *Digestive System* takes in a variety of liquid and solid foods, breaks it down into useful enzymes and extracts its useful nutrients in appropriate volumes. Unwanted wastes are removed from your body as stools, urine, perspiration or dyspeptic gas (fart or burp). Your *Nervous System* receives and routes the control signals from the brain to activate the proper muscles and organs as it responds to internal and external stimuli—like when the *Muscular System* manipulates locomotion, facial expressions, coughing or sneezing, etc. or as a reaction to its environment. Other structures or functions that complement these systems include the *Immune, Reproductive, Skeletal, Endocrine and Integumentary Systems*. The *Brain* is the command center of all these disparate but interlinked functions. It assimilates outside stimuli like danger, fear, emotions, impulses (fight or flight)—processes and prepares the affected organs to receive instant orders (relayed through the nervous system) to react accordingly. It is the ultimate computer.

It will not be necessary for our purpose here, to expand details about them, but just to skim over their various participations as it affects our overall well being. This is being included to emphasize the need in preparing your body properly as you go about doing your various tasks for the day. Proper breathing for at least 3-5 minutes upon waking up, or before embarking upon any kind of exercise or rigorous activity, helps prepare your bodily systems to perform more efficiently.

Now, on to your exercise. It starts when the alarm clock wakes you up!

Chapter IV

BED EXERCISES FOR SENIORS AND THE LAZY MAN!

I. *BREATHING FUNDAMENTALS* (For Beginners)

Even *before* you open your eyes, you *must* start your 3-5 minutes of *Breathing Fundamentals* by performing the following:

1. While lying supine in bed, *eyes closed*, raise and rest both arms limply atop the bed and over your head, forming a U-shape with the wrists near, but not touching the ears, open palms, facing up.

2. THUMBS LOCK DOWN (TLD)—With all five fingers of both hands extended upwards, curl both *index fingers* downwards, touching your palm, press your thumbs down firmly over it, with the rest of the fingers (middle, ring and little fingers) straight up. This position is maintained throughout some of the legs, arms and finger exercises, ostensibly to help retain the bio-energy forces within the system.

3. INHALE SLOWLY (INH) through the nose (mouth closed) for *10 seconds*; coursing the air through the back of your neck and lungs, (while you pull your belly muscles inward), forcing it down to the bottom of your lungs, then

4. HOLD IT THERE AND PRESS IT DOWN (HDP)—(you do this by grunting abruptly the word "UNGH") holding your breath for *25 seconds* (Note: should the allotted 25 seconds be not enough when performing your exercise regimen, INHALE QUICKLY ONCE (*Do Not Exhale*) until your exercise routine is done.)

5. EXHALE SLOWLY (EXH) for *12 Seconds* through gritted teeth (first exhale through the mouth; the rest shall be made through the nose).

The foregoing Breathing Regimen is known as the 10-25-12 Exercise Beat! Resume normal breathing sequence for the next 20 Seconds, then re-start the Exercise Beat and repeat process for 3-5 minutes. (Note: When starting off on this Breathing Dynamics, it is recommended that you pause for 20 seconds before resuming the next phase). Both INHALING and EXHALING actions should be performed *gradually in the suggested time frame.*

You MUST be able to master or perfect these BREATHING FUNDAMENTALS as a condition in performing the rest of your Exercise Regimen. This is required, specially the portion where you HOLD YOUR BREATH (by abruptly grunting the word "UNGH" and *holding your breath at the bottom of your lungs* for *25 minutes while performing your Aerobics Exercises.* It gets easier with practice.

Chapter V

II. *LIMBERING—UP ROUTINES (See accompanying Line Art Illustrations)*

Having performed your 3-5 minutes Breathing Exercise, *do not get up from bed yet*. Proceed to THUMBS LOCK—DOWN MODE (TLD).

THUMBS LOCK—DOWN MODE (TLD)—lower both arms limply beside your body, curl both index fingers lightly inwards, gently pressing them downwards with your thumbs to your palms, with the rest of your fingers pointing outwards and holding it steady in that position.

1. EYEBALLS EXERCISES—(INH; HDP & TLD) slowly open your eyes, gradually lower (for 3-seconds count) your sights or eyeballs *downwards* to the directions of your feet; then move it slowly *upwards* towards the direction of your forehead. Still with your head held steady in place, slowly redirect your eyeballs to the *left*, then to the *right*. Then slowly *rotate* your eyeballs *Clockwise*, then *Counterclockwise* (The foregoing exercises must be performed only once and done while HOLDING YOR BREATH for 25 seconds or more as needed—(*See accompanying Line Art illustrations*), and then SLOWLY (for 12 Seconds) EXHALE (EXH).

C A U T I O N: When performing the rest of the Legs, Arms, and other Routines, you are encouraged to start off easy (A).

Beginners are encouraged to gradually perform these routines in the ascending ORDER OF PROFECIENCY by repeating the exercise regimen as follows:

A) BASIC ROUTINE (10-20-12 Secs. Beat—*F I V E (5) TIMES*

B) INTERMEDIATE (12-25-14 Secs. Beat—*S E V E N (7) TIMES*

C) ADVANCED (12-30-16 Secs. Beat—*N I N E (9) TIMES*

Always be mindful that these exercises *must* be performed while AIR IS ON HOLD (HDP) at the bottom of your lungs and index fingers on *lock-down* mode. If the 20-30 Seconds period is not sufficient to complete your exercise segment, you may INHALE once, but *not exhale*, until you finish the routine.

2. FEET & LEGS ROUTINES—(For beginners)

a) **Toes Curl—(INH; HDP & TLD)** With both arms resting limply on your sides, body supine, slowly (for the 3-seconds count) **curl all toes all the way downward, then upwards.** Repeat process for 4 more times, then **(EXH).** Open up your palms and resume regular breathing for 20 seconds.

b) **Foot Curls—(INH; HDP; TLD)** With the usual 3-seconds count, (with both heels on stationary points), slowly bend both feet **downwards,** then **upwards.** Repeat process 4 more times, then SLOWLY **(EXH).** Open up your palms and resume regular breathing for 20 seconds.

c) **Foot Twists—(INH; HDP; TLD)** With both heels on stationary pivot, slowly (3-seconds count) **Twist both heels extremely outwards, then inwards crossing right foot atop the other in an "X"** position, then repeat outward twist. On next inward twist, alternately fan right foot to be under left sole of your palms and vice-versa, then resume regular breathing for 20 seconds.

d) **Leg Rotations—(INH; HDP' TLD)** with left leg supporting, slowly lift up your right leg upwards; upon reaching its apex, **Rotate** it slowly **Counterclockwise,** then **Clockwise** then lower it slowly. Now with right leg supporting, lift up **Left leg slowly,** then Rotate it **Counterclockwise,** then **clockwise,** lower left leg and SLOWLY **(EXH)**. Open up your palms your palms and resume regular breathing for 20 seconds.

e) **Military Split—(INH; HDP; TLD)** with both arms supporting, slowly raise both legs upwards, then upon reaching the apex, slowly **split** up both legs **sideward in midair** away from each other, then while still **suspended, slowly return both legs** back to its center position about 6 inches apart without touching each other; then lower them down, and **without touching the bed's surface, raise** both legs upwards again, repeating process once more. On 3rd & 4th process, alternately cross both legs in mid-air forming an "X" twice, and gradually lower them downwards and SLOWLY **(EXH)**. Open up both palms and resume regular breathing pace for 20 seconds.

f) **Spine & Body Lifts—(INH; HDP; TLD)** With both arms supporting, bend knees upwards, feet sliding flat toward buttocks, and with both heels and head as **pivots**, raise entire torso upwards, then slowly lower body down and without touching the bed, raise it once more. On the 3rd and 4th sequence, with torso still suspended in mid-air, **rock body up and down twice**, then lower body downwards to resting position and SLOWLY **(EXH)**. Open both palms and resume regular breathing pace for 20 seconds.

Chapter VI

III. SYSTEM'S RESTORATION REGIMEN

After the foregoing limbering up routines (Feet & Legs), it will be necessary to *cool down* your muscles and respiratory systems before embarking on your next exercise regimen. This is accomplished by reverting back to a relaxing sequence of deep breathing fundamentals, hence:

    a. THUMBS IN LOCK DOWN POSITION (TLD)—With *all* five fingers pointing upwards, *curl* both *index* fingers downwards touching your palms and press it gently down with both thumbs.

    b. INHALE (INH) Slowly for 10 Seconds (again coursing air to flow through the nose, the back of your neck and through the back of your lungs, your stomach pressed inwards, well until air is directed to the bottom of your lungs when you grunt the word; "UNGH", then

    c. HOLD AIR DOWN AND PRESS (HDP) for 25 seconds, after which

    d. EXHALE SLOWLY (EXH) for 12 Seconds, then *resume* regular breathing pace for another 20 seconds.

N O T E:

    1. For BEGINNERS, the Breathing Sequence in this Restoration regimen is *(10-25-12)* where EXHALING (EXH) takes a bit longer to give more time for your system to effectively start off the disposal mechanisms of your body's wastes.

2. For the REGULAR OR ADVANCED Breathing Cycles, the following sequences are advised:

BREATHING FUNDAMENTALS (12-30-15) Beat!

RESTORATION REGIMEN (10-25-12) Beat

Chapter VII

FIRST LEVEL (FUNDAMENTAL) PROFECIENCY EXERCISES

IV. *ARMS & FINGERS ROUTINE*. (Note: PROFECIENCY ROUTINES Composed of the BASIC, INTERMEDIATE & ADVANCED SYSTEMS and by Integrating holding your breath with 20, 25 & 30 SECONDS Breathing Cycles)

a. FINGERS OPEN/CLOSE ROUTINE—(INH *10 seconds*; HDP *25 Seconds*) with both arms spread-eagled flat to the sides (like a cross), palms facing up, alternately Open and close the fingers of both palms *one by one*, holding your fingers tightly inwards for 3 seconds, abruptly spring it open outwards, then slowly (for another 3-seconds count) compressed them inwards again, repeating process 4 more times, then (EXH-*12 Seconds*).

b. CROSS ARMS ROUTINE—(INH; HDP; TLD) Raise both arms upward towards the ceiling, then swing both arms inwards, one arm atop the other, forming a big letter "X", then spread both arms away from each other about 30 degrees higher to the sides, then crossing them again to the center alternately (this time the other arm atop) to the 3-seconds count, repeating this process 4 more times, then spread-eagle again both arms to rest on the sides, open both palms and then, (EXH) and resume 20-minute normal breathing pace.

c. ELBOW ROTATIONS—With fingers on both hands forming a big letter "C", anchor finger tips atop both shoulders, raising both elbows to shoulder levels. (INH), (HDP) Rotate both extended elbows Counterclockwise for the 3-seconds count for Five times, then while still holding your breath, rotate them Clockwise for also five times. Resume 20-seconds breathing pace.

d. CIRCULAR ARMS FLAIL ROUTINE—(INH; HDP; TLD) With the left hand resting on the side, raise right arm to the topmost level, trace a big letter "O" 3 times with it Counterclockwise to the 3-seconds count, then reverse it Clockwise for 3 times also. Lower right arm, then raise left arm and perform the same routine. Repeat both Arms Flail 4 more times, then (EXC), open both palms and resume regular breathing pace.

e. DOUBLE ARMS SIDE FLAIL ROUTINE—(INH; HDP, TLD) Raise both arms to the center, a foot apart; swing both arms together to the extreme right slowly to the 3-seconds count (Maintaining the same distance apart), then to the left. Repeat left & right flail routines 4 more times, then (EXH) and resume regular 20-seconds breathing pace.

f. TORSO SCRAPE—Interlace fingers with both thumbs pressing lightly against each other, palms open and facing towards the feet. Lower conjoined palms to the bottom (but not touching) the chin, then (INH; HDP) move both palms steadily downwards tracing the surface of your torso without actually touching it, abruptly stop atop your groin, then raise and separate both palms sideward; re-clasp both fingers plunging them again to your lower chin and tracing the same surface contour of your breast and abdomen downwards, repeating this process 4 m ore times, then (EXH) and resume regular 20-seconds breathing pace, both arms resting spread-eagled on both sides. Get down from your bed and proceed to perform the

Chapter VIII

SECOND-LEVEL (INTERMEDIATE) PROFECIENCY EXERCISES.

V. *WARM-UP EXERCISES*. Ideally, this could be performed with bare feet touching the ground, grass or floor having free air circulation. Start-up position is with both hands akimbo beside the waist, feet 18 inches apart and firmly planted on the ground. In this position, start your BREATHING REGIMEN (INH—12 seconds; HDP 30 seconds; EXH 10 SECDONDS) or the Breathing Fundamentals of *12-30-15*. Repeat Breathing sequences for 4 more times, then Resume regular breathing pace for the next 20 Seconds and commence your Warm-Up Exercises.

   a. FORWARD ARMS THRUST—move left foot 18 inches to the side, Interlace all four fingers (except thumbs) and thrust conjoined palms facing outward on horizontal level; then (INH;HDP) grind hips counterclockwise in a circular motion for 8 times, then reverse grinding movement for also 8 times; lower both arms loosely to the sides, then (EXH). Resume regular breathing pace for 20 seconds.

   b. OVERHEAD ARMS THRUST—From start-up position, Interlace fingers of both palms in front of you as before, reverse conjoined palms outwards as you raise them both directly overhead, (INH; HDP) grind hips Counterclockwise in a circular motion for 8 times, then reverse grinding to clockwise motion for also 8 times, unclasp hands, lower both arms to the sides and (EXH). Resume regular 20-seconds breathing pace.

   c. BACKHAND CLASP ARMS THRUST—Place both hands behind your back (not touching it), right palms facing up and with left palm facing down, clasp all four fingers tightly in a vise-like grip and with interlinked hands 2 inches away from your back (INH; HDP), grind your hips around Counterclockwise for 9 times, reverse direction for Clockwise, 8 more times, unclasp fingers and drop hands to the sides, then (EXH). Resume regular 20-seconds breathing pace.

d. STATIONARY JOGGING—(INH), (HDP), (TLD)—Perform jogging-in-place at a comfortable clip (say 45 seconds), then open up fingers and (EXH) slowly as you resume the usual 20-seconds normal breathing pace.

Chapter IX

THIRD LEVEL (ADVANCED) PROFECIENCY EXERCISES:

(KNEE BENDS, BODY TWISTS, TWIRLS AND HAND SCRAPES)
(See Line Art Illustrations)

    a   KNEE BENDS—With feet on Start-up position (18" apart), place both hands akimbo to the hips, then (INH; HDP 12-30-16) and perform Knee Bends for 8 times, then (EXH). Resume 20-seconds regular breathing break.

    b.   BODY TWISTS—from start-up position, feet 18 inches apart, place both arms to the sides vertically on shoulder's level (like a cross), (INH; HDP) Twist your shoulders and arms Clockwise intermittently to the extreme right, pause, then reverse to twist your shoulders, arms and entire upper torso extremely to the left in an intermittent and jerky movement, repeating alternate Body Twists for 8 times, then (EXH). Drop both arms to the sides and resume 20-seconds regular breathing pace.

    c.   BODY TWIRL—Raise both arms upward 45 degrees to the sides, (INH;HDP) with your left heel as pivot, toes raised upwards, propel your body around counterclockwise with your right foot with both arms freely flailing naturally sideward as you turn; (HINT: as you turn, keep your head steady and focus your OPEN eyes steady upon a fixed point on the wall for a time before you permit your head to follow the turn, but quickly revert back to the same imaginary point on the wall at a little above eye level. DO NOT CLOSE YOUR EYES while your body is turning and don't look down). Continue Body twirl for 8 Counts, then drop both arms to the sides and (EXH). Continue to gaze at that imaginary fixed point above eye-level on the wall as you resume 20-seconds regular breathing pace. From start-up position, arms raised 45 degrees to the sides (INH;HDP) and with your right heel as pivot, propel your body Clockwise, (head steady, eyes focused on imaginary and stationary point on the wall above eye-level) and repeat process for 8 more times. Stop and continue to focus your open eyes upon the same stationary point on the wall as you lower both arms to the sides and (EXH). Resume regular 20-seconds breathing pace. This exercise is to help stabilize your balance and prevent Vertigo.

d. FINGER FLAIL & HEAD TURN—While doing regular breathing, raise both arms 45 degrees from the elbow to the front, shake both hands from limp wrists repeatedly for 12 times (as if shaking away waters from your fingers). Place your arms akimbo on your hips and with torso and both feet steady, slowly rotate or twist your head to the extreme right, then to extreme left. You will hear some nerves or muscles snap and crackle as it loosens up. Repeat process 2 more times, this time nodding your head alternately up and down.

e. FULL ARMS AND BODY SCRAPE—From start-up position, raise your Left arm to a 45 degree angle. With your right thumb and forefinger, form a big half circle (like a letter "C") and bring it atop your left shoulder without touching it, then gradually slide it downwards (lightly brushing parts of your arm) all the way to the tips of your left fingers and flail your open right palm three times outwards (as if shaking away waters from your hands). Repeat process 3 times to cover all sides of the arm. Then, lift your right arm forward (45 degrees from elbow) and with your left fingers forming a big letter "C), scrape the right arm from the upper shoulder, all the way down to the tips of your right open palms, then shake off your open left hand loosely 3 times.

f. TORSO AND LEG SCRAPES—From start-up position, raise both open palms to center level, facing down, finger tips abutting in front of the upper front shoulders and scrape it downwards,(as if removing water droplets from your body), all the way to your thighs (and when possible) to your feet, returning your open palms to the upper shoulder and scrapping downwards all parts of your body from the top, and downwards to the front, sides and back of your legs and feet again, as if scraping imaginary water droplets from all around your body. Repeat process once and raise both palms 45 degrees outwards and shake it vigorously loose 12 times alternately scraping of imaginary water droplets from your front, sides and back of your palms. This action is said to remove the negative emanations from around your body, legs and hands after performing this Exercise regimen.

Chapter X

LINE ARTS ILLUSTRATIONS

Body Posture—When seated, the LOTUS position is most ideal. For Seniors and those ailing, they can sit in a 4 legged chair, with their back held straight 4 inches from the chair's back. Legs must be crossed at the ankles, biceps held loose and 2 inches from the body with the forearms held parallel to the floor with wrists and palms up.

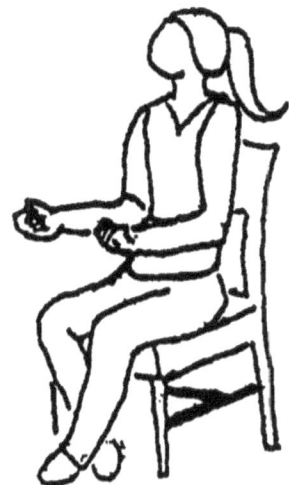

Lock mode is when the thumb is placed gently across the palm of the hand with the thumb curls softly over the index finger

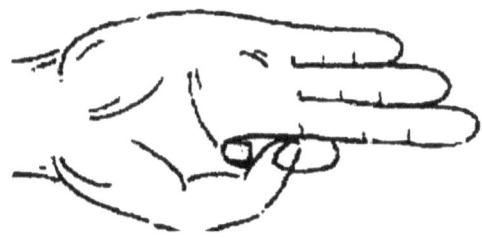

While doing the BREATHING EXERCISES your spine must remain straight. Remove all distractions from your mind by concentrating on a point in the middle area behind your neck.

BREATHING SEQUENCE (THE ARCEBUCHE METHOD)

INHALING (INH)—Breath air slowly through your nose for *15 seconds*. Pull air uninterrupted into the back of your lungs, by passing the air through the back of your neck.

HOLD BREATH AND PRESS IT DOWNLOAD (HPD)—
With the air at the bottom of your lungs, PRESS IT DOWN IN ONE ABRUPT THRUST AND HOLD IT FOR *30 SECONDS*. This is when you will perform your exercises.

EXHALING (EXH)—Proceed to release air slowly for 12 seconds through the nose. Note: On the first release, exhale through gritted teeth, thereafter, all exhaling must be done through the nose.

It is important that you attain perfection in this exercise. Remember the timing sequence (INHALE—5 seconds; HOLD DOWN AND PRESS—30 seconds; EXHALING—12 seconds or 15-20. For beginners, start with a 10-15-12 sequence and practice this breathing techniques 2-3 times a day. Remember to stay in the correct body position stated before.

LIMBERING-UP ROUTINES

You start your day when you wake up in bed. Do not get up. *Start by doing a 3 minute Breathing Exercise,* then perform the following:

EYEBALL EXERCISES—(INH;HDP) Open eyes and slowly look down at your feet. Slowly move your eyeballs to look upward to the top of your head. Look to your extreme left, then to your extreme right. Rotate eyeballs counterclockwise once, then clockwise once. Do this only once. (EXH)

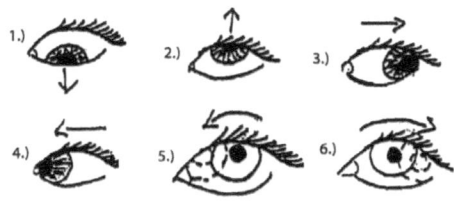

FEET &LEGS ROUTINE

Toe curl—(INH;HDP) Laying down on your back with both arms resting at sides in Lock-up mode, for a 3 second curl all toes downwards, then upwards; repeat the process 3 times while holding 20-second breathe then (EXH).

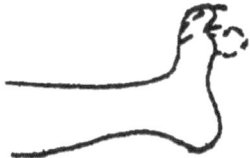

Feet Curl—(INH;HDP) With the usual 3 second count, slowly move feet downward, then upward. Repeat this process three times, then (EXH).

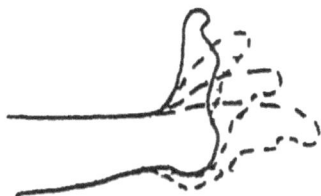

Leg Lifts—(INH;HDP) With the right leg supporting, lift left leg slowly upward to a 45 degree angle, hold it stationary for at least 2 seconds, then lower it slowly. Repeat the sequence alternating between right and left legs three times per leg, then (EXH).

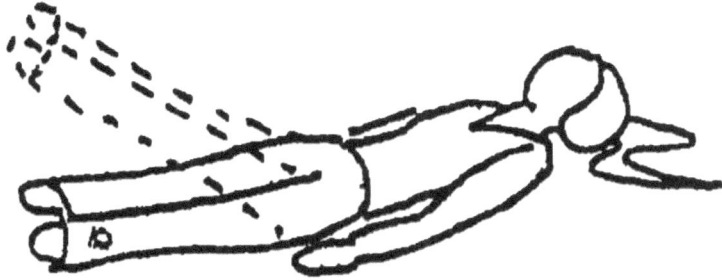

Leg Rotations—(INH;HDP) With the right leg supporting, lift left leg slowly upward to a 45 degree angle, rotate it counterclockwise for a 3-second count, then clockwise and slowly lower it. Do the same for the right, alternating both feet for three times each, then (EXH).

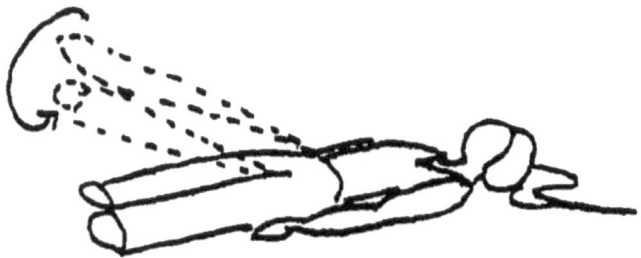

Military Split—(INH;HDP) With both arms supporting, raise both legs slowly, then spilt them sideways in mid-air (three to five times in 3-second count), lower both feet slowly, then (EXH).

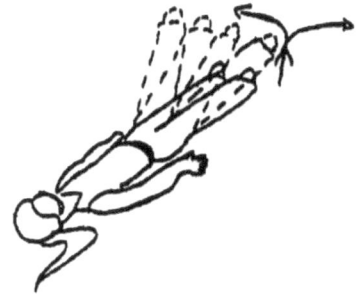

Spine and Body Lift—(INH;HDP) With both arms supporting, bend both knees upwards, with both heels and head supporting, lift entire torso upwards and while suspended, slowly rock it up and down for a 3-second count, repeat rocking movement three more times, slowly moving torso, flatten both legs back to original position, then (EXH).

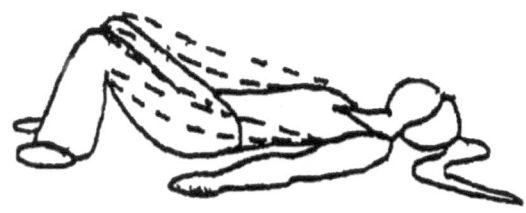

ARMS AND FINGERS ROUTINE

Fingers close/Open Routine—(INH ;HDP) With both arms spread eagled to sides, alternately Close and Open fingers to the 3-second count 5 times, then (EXH).

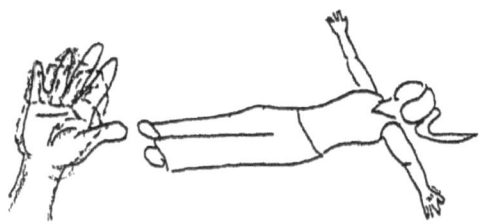

Cross Arms Routine—(INH;HDP) With fingers in Lock-up mode, swing both arms toward your center breast forming an "X" swing back to sides for the 3-second count, one arm alternately over the other 5 times each arm, then (EXH).

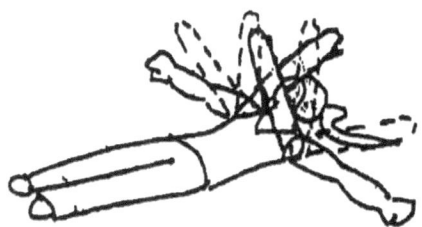

Circular Flail Arms Routine—(INH;HDP) With fingers in Lock-up mode, raise right arm upwards, with your clichéd fist, trace a big "O" counterclockwise three times for the usual 3-second count, lower it to side, then lift again, tracing the "O" clockwise three times; lower arm. Raise left arm and repeat process three times on each arm (EXH).

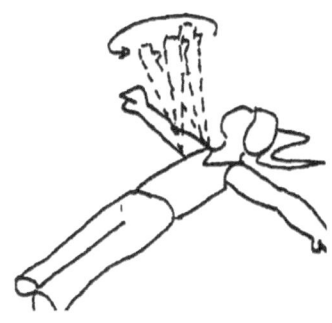

GET DOWN FROM BED AND START UP YOUR WARM UP EXERCISES

Forward Arms Thrust—(INH; HDP) Move left foot 18 inches to side, interlace fingers, then thrust both arms forward with palms facing away from body. Grind hips counterclockwise to the usual 3-second beat for 9 counts, lower both arms to sides and bring left foot back to center, then (EXH). Interlace fingers, then thrust both arms forward with palms facing out then (INH;HDP) grind hips clockwise for 9 counts, lower both arms to sides, return left foot to center, then (EXH).

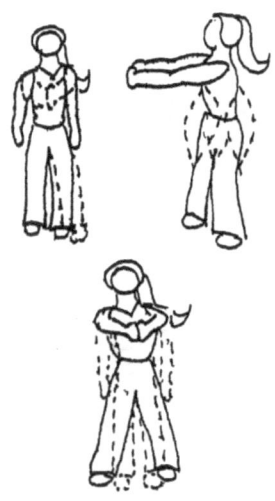

Double Arms Side Flail Routine—(INH; HDP) With both hands in Lock-up mode, bring both arms upward to center, a foot apart. Swing them both to right side twice stopping at center to the usual 3-second count, then to the left side twice. Repeat process 5 times, then (EXH). Flail your palms rapidly up and down for 5 times.

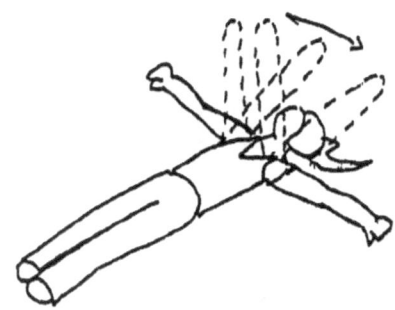

Front Torso Scrape—(INH; HDP) Interlacing both hands with thumb tips touching, place hands an inch over your forehead and begin moving it down in a scraping motion towards your groin, passing one inch over your breast and stomach and abruptly lift it upwards, repeating process for 9 counts, then (EXH).

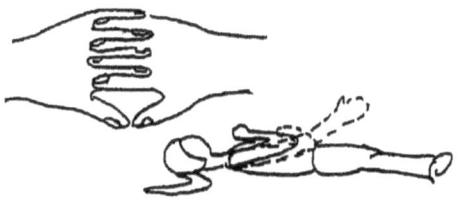

Overhead Arms Thrust—Move right foot 18 inches away, interlace hands and thrust arms directly overhead with palms facing up. (INH: HDP) grind hips counterclockwise for 9 times, return both arms to sides, then (EXH). Interlace arms again, thrust arms directly overhead with palms facing up and grind hips clockwise for 9 times, lower both arms, return right foot to center position, then (EXH).

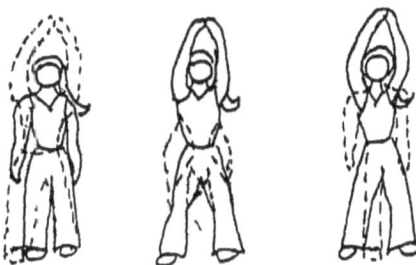

Behind Back Arms Thrust—Move right foot 18 inches away interlace hands behind back holding hands 4 inches from body, (INH; HDP) grind hips counterclockwise for 9 times, bring arms back to side, then (EXH). Interlace hands behind back again (INH;HDP) grind hips clockwise for 9 times, lower arms, bring left foot back to center, then (EXH).

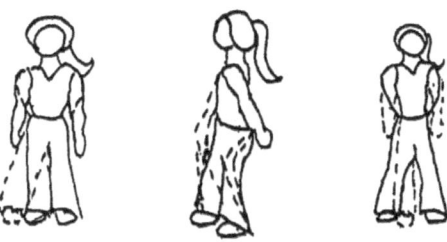

Knee bends—Interlace fingers, invert palms outwards and extend both arms forward, then (INH;HDP) and start knee bends for 9 count, then (EXH).

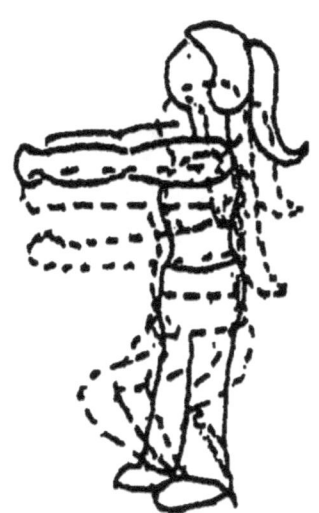

Flail both arms loosely on the sides clockwise, then counterclockwise for 3 times. Then clockwise for 3times, then proceed to the **Cooling Down Routine**.

WRIST STRETCHING EXERCISES PERMITS BETTER BLOOD FLOW WHILE STRENGTHENING YOUR FINGER JOINTS, HANDS, MUSCLES, AND SHOULDERS

Wrist exercise is performed when you drop down to to the floor, (as if starting to do push-ups) but instead of supporting your body weight with both both palms, SPREAD OUT ALL FINGERS of both hands, with only the FINGERTIPS touching the floor to support your entire body weight. Then perform a few PUSH-UPS, using again the 10-25-12 seconds Exercise Beat, performing it while under HDP in the following regimen:

a) BASIC or INTRODUCTORY - Five (5) Times
b) INTERMEDIATE- Seven (7) Times
c) ADVANCE - Nine (9) Times

Chapter XI

VI. *SYSTEM'S RESTORATION OR COOLING DOWN PHASE*

After performing any form of rigorous exercise, it is always advisable to restore your system's metabolism gradually before embarking on the day's regular activities. This is required to help return your systems into standby or resting mode. This transition is needed to prevent abrupt changes, which can impair the reaction profile of your finely tuned system. Consider when you expose yourself abruptly to extreme heat or cold temperatures, or jumping from the second floor of your house without using the stairway. Cooling-down regimen as the 'stairway' towards bodily normalization.

The 10-25-12 Breathing Sequence.

Find a comfortable chair, sit straight, with your back at least 4 inches away from the backrest, close your eyes, concentrate your thoughts upon a fixed point behind your nape and with open palms resting limply atop your thighs, commence to perform the following:

1. INHALE (INH) slowly for 10 seconds.

2. HOLD YOUR BREATH AND PRESS IT DOWN (HDP) FOR 25 seconds.

3. EXHALE (EXH) for 12 seconds, then resume regular breathing break for 20 seconds.

4. Repeat breathing sequence (10-25-12) for the next 5 minutes, open your eyes slowly. Stand up, stretch & shake your wrists and body loosely for a few times, swivel your head around TWICE, Clockwise & Counterclockwise. Crackling

sounds may be heard from your neck muscles and cartilages. When you begin to feel refreshed & not tired, (even after the exercise), you've just successfully completed your regimen, my friend. CONGRATULATIONS!

Chapter XII

FINGER EXERCISES (MUDRAS)

No. 1—GYAN MUDRA (KNOWLEDGE)

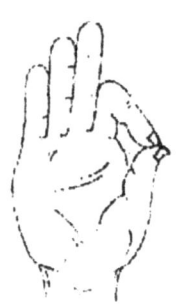

METHOD: Touch the tips of the Index finger and thumb With the other three fingers stretched out and press lightly. These are the sites of the pituitary and endocrine glands. It enhances memory and sharpens the brain. Said to help prevent insomnia and other psychological disorders.

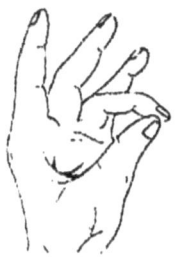

No. 2—PRITHVI MUDRA—(EARTH)

The tip of the ring finger should touch the lip of the thumb with the rest of the other fingers stretched outwards. Said to help increase weight and makes skin glow.

No. 3—VARUNA MUDRA (WATER)

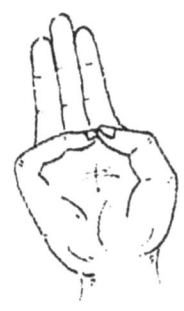

Let the tip off the little finger touch the lip of the thumb as the three fingers are stretched out. Said to help retain blood clarity by balancing its water content. Prevents muscle shrinkage and gastroenteritis pain.

No. 4—VUYA MUDRA (AIR)

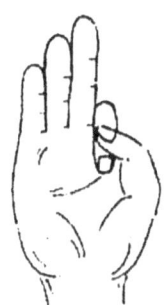

Curl the index finger downwards to your palm and press it lightly with your thumb, while the rest of the three fingers are held straight up. Said to help cure rheumatism, arthritis, gout and Parkinson's disease. Useful for cervical spondelytis paralysis to face and catching of nerves in the neck. Correct gas disorder in the stomach.

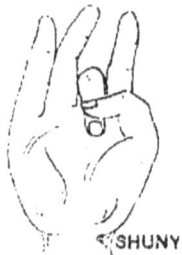

No. 5—SHUNYA MUDRA (EMPTINESS)

Cut the middle finger down to palm and press it lightly with the thumb, the rest of the fingers stretched upwards. Said to help alleviate earaches, while deemed useful for the hearing impaired and the mentally-challenged.

No. 6—SURYA MUDRA (SUNO)

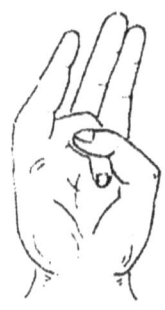

Ring finger should be bent down towards the palm and gently presses it with the thumb while the other fingers are stretched upwards. Said to help reduce cholesterol, anxiety, weight, and indigestion problems.

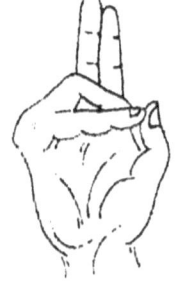

No. 7—PRANA MUDRA (LIFE)

Bend the little finger and ring finger to the tip of the thumb, with the rest of the two fingers stretched upwards. Said to help reduce eye-related ailments, reduce fatigue and vitamin deficiency.

No. 8—APAN MUDRA (DIGESTION)

Tips of the middle and ring fingers should be bent downwards to touch the palm with the thumb pressing it down and other two fingers stretched upwards. Said to help alleviate diabetes, constipation and bowel movement.

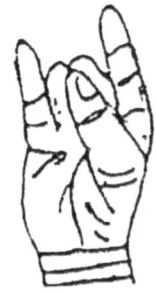

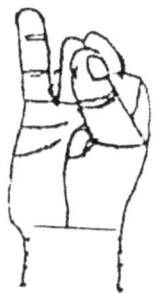

No. 9—APANA VAYU MUDRA (HEART)

The middle and ring finger tips touches the tip of the thumb, as the index finger touches the base of the thumb, the little finger stretched upward. Helps regularize heart beat, bowel movement and gastric problems.

No. 10—LINGA MUDRA (HEAT & ENERGY)

Interlace both fingers of both hands, keeping the thumb of the left hand vertically straight upward, encircle it with the index finger and the thumb of the right hand. Said to help give power to the lungs, reduce phlegm, bronchial infections and invigorates the body.

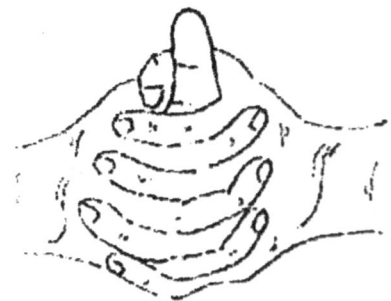

Chapter XIII

OTHER SUGGESTED HEALTH PRACTICES

1. Every morning when you wake up, or after performing your Light Aerobics exercise **drink two glassful of water** at room temperature. This helps wash away the toxins accumulated during the night.

2. Before sleeping, gargle with a **pure strength mouthwash** like Citrus-flavored Listerin , etc. to help ward off colds and influenza. Do the same when you wake up.

3. Before each regular meal, eat a small serving of **fresh fruit or salad**. Your stomach will start producing gastric juices to help hasten digestion. Take just one full meal a day and take more light snacks or healthy foods.

4. Sea foods like mackerel, salmon, tuna, etc. has **Omega 3** fats beneficial to your body. Gray-colored Salmon are ocean-sourced and preferable to the pink-colored or farm-raised Salmon. Baked fish are healthier when taken with two spoonful of **Spanish Extra Virgin Oil**. Frying is discouraged.

5. If possible, acquire a **separate refrigerator** and load it with health foods.

6. **Morning sunshine** up to 10:00 AM is a great source of Vitamin D.

7. On your bedroom or bathroom door jambs, request a carpenter to install a two-inch round bar or tube whre you can perform periodic **chinning bar exercises** to help loosen up joints and tune your muscles.

8. Take dietary food **supplements** to help reinforce your nutrition deficiencies. Fresh and natural fruits or vegetables are great sources of healthy foods.

9. A spoonful of **raw oatmeal or a glassful of pure grape. strawberry, orange, apple, beet or carrot juices** or a combination of them is said to help lower bad cholesterol levels and even found to ward off cancer. Buy a **Juicer machine** and drink a combination of these healing foods at least once a week. It will help alleviate many ailments and may even prevent the onset of dreaded diseases.

10. After bowel movements, wipe off your butt with dry tissues (twice) and wet a portion of folded tissues (1/3) and wipe your butt with them, following it with dry tissues. Wash your hands with Soap and water, always after using the bathroom.

11. **"ALKALINE WATER"**—Cut 2-3 thin slices of lemon, place it in a cup or glass and add drinking water. Drink it for the whole day and keep on adding water. This is said to help ward off a number of cancer—destroying malignant cells for 12 types of cancerous ailments including colon, breast, prostate, lung, pancreas, etc.

12. **Mosquitos** and other evening bugs are bothersome pests—specially when you and your guests wishes to spend an evening outdoors. Spray the surrounding areas and lawn with **Listerine** and around your seats. Watch them disappear!

13. **A hoarse voice** can be cured overnight! Make three thins slices of **Fresh Ginger** and deposit one every hour on top of your tongue (don't chew it), the third slice, before going to sleep. Your voice will be restored the following morning!

14. **Gout** makes you suffer and irritable. Eat six **Fresh Cherry Fruits** a **day for a week** and relief may be enjoyed within the week. You can also drink **Cherry Juice** (black or red Cherry) and dilute it with equal amount of water.

15. **Diabetes** may be tamed by eating **bitter melon or bitter gourd** (Filipinos call it **Ampalaya** or its Spanish name **Amarigoso**). These are available from Filipino or Asian Stores. Take a couple of this fruit (6 to 8 inches long), slice it lengthwise, remove the pith and make thin slices across—One Eight of an inch. As a salad, marinate it overnight in one cup vinegar, half a cup of water and two spoonfuls of sugar. It can be combined with other fruits for juicing or you can use a blender. You can also take the whole vine plant, stems, leaves, fruits and all, chopped it fine, dry under the sun and boil until water is just one fourth of original volume, colored black, refrigerate and drink portions of it as tea or a cup a day.

16. **Dizzy Spells** and Nausea are often results of low blood pressure. This occurs when you stand up abruptly. Try eating a few servings of **Chicken or Pork Liver a week**. Alternate it with a couple of Hard Boiled Eggs, eat only the **Egg Whites!**. Relief could come within days.

17. **COFFEE—3 Tricks to Make it Superhealthy**

    Mike Geary, a Certified Nutritionist Specialist and Personal Trainer *help-desk@truthabout abs.com*, suggested the following:

    1. Avoid Adding refined sugar or artificial sweeteners to your Coffee. Use a small touch of organic **Maple Syrup** or a half packet of **Natural Stevia.**
    2. Avoid natural Creamers, liquid or power, but use **organic grass-feed cream** or **coconut milk/cream.**
    3. Load your coffee with more **anti-oxidants** to make it tastier, like **cinnamon** to help control blood sugar.

18. When you take a **Warm Shower** and, as you're about to finish, turn the water to as hot you can stand for the last **two minutes**, then abruptly turn the temperature down to as Cold as you can. Scandinavians, immediately after their Sauna Baths, immediately Plunge into the icy waters to help

jolt your bodily systems and revitalize blood circulation. Now, being a lazy man, my version of a cold bath ending, is to make a complete turn under a cold spray clockwise and another complete 180 degree turn, counter-clockwise.

19. Think of **happy and positive thoughts**. Feel-good brain agents like Dopamine and Serotonin are secreted in your brain in reaction to stimuli. Depressing thoughts or Situations causes stress. Take a bigger picture of life like the many blessings you enjoy. You're not sick, blind, homeless, in a hospital or in prison.

20. Your body is a **well-oiled machine!**. It will respond with the manner in which you operate or maintain it. Its inherent self-healing properties are better enhanced with proper diet, breathing, exercise and a healthier life style. It will deteriorate conversely should you embrace habitually those that make your body lower its guards. Other than your physician, you are the best source of your own bio-feedback mechanisms—be it mental, physical or psychological. Learn more and trust your own body.

Chapter XIV

BENEFICIAL EFFECTS OF PROPER BREATHING MAY BE OBTAINED WHEN

1. You feel sleepy, sluggish or lethargic.
2. You have headaches or other bodily or muscular pains.
3. Feeling tired or morose.
4. In search of ideas, concepts or solutions.
5. Before making a presentation or speech.
6. Making a letter or responding to one.
7. In the midst of discussions, argumentations or debates.
8. You feel "down" and require emotional "lift".
9. Feeling of physical and/or emotional debility.
10. Before & after sex
11. Before embarking on a long drive or activity.
12. Needs a 'waker-upper" in between activities.
13. Convalescing or before taking medicines.
14. Upon waking up, before exercises or "cooling down".
15. Before going on sports activities.
16. You feel like "recharging" your system after sedentary periods like watching TV, reading, solving puzzle, long trips, meditations, classes, etc.
17. After a long and stressful day, when angry, irritated, fearful, or after receiving 'bad news" or general feeling of unease.
18. A need for increased alertness and invigoration.

How your body reacts and benefit from this Breathing Regimen will largely depend upon the level of practice and proficiency you manage to attain. When feeling buoyant and relaxed after breathing or cooling-down sessions, your body is now responding to the benefits of a more oxygenated system. Include a moderate or healthier lifestyle and proper diet, makes for a more vibrant and fulfilled living. To reiterate my earlier view, we only get one change for life in this world. Let's not botch it with foolish choices. The quality on how we spend the rest of our days will ultimately depend upon how we nourish and nurture the very system that makes it all possible—our human body. *If we take proper care of it, it will take care of us. Let's breathe properly, live the proper Lifestyle anti be happy for the rest of our days!*

Chapter XV

SUGGESTED FOOD AND NUTRITION REMINDERS

The purpose of this section is to serve as a helpful adjunct to the preceding exercise regimen. It is in no way designed to make the reader experts or authorities on nutrition. For more detailed information on this subject, it is always advisable to contact your physician.

For our purpose, we will just skim through the more relevant portions on this subject. To start off, let us try to understand what the term "Nutrition" is all about. In a book entitled "Nutrition and Physical Fitness: by Bogert, Briggs and Calloway, (Published by W. B. Saunders Company), the authors defined Nutrition as *the science of food as it relates to the optimal health and performance.* The food we ingest contain some 45 important substances generally called *nutrients.* They may be grouped into six general classes:

1. Carbohydrates
2. Fats
3. Proteins
4. Vitamins
5. Minerals
6. Water

Carbohydrates, fats and proteins are often grouped as *Fuel or Energy* nutrients, used by the body to supply energy and heat. *Proteins, minerals and water* are used for building new tissues and repairing damaged ones. *Mineral salts and Vitamins* acts as body regulators to help stabilize the functions of nerves, muscles and other bodily roles.

Lest we get sidetracked into the more technical details of nutrition, let us visit the more relevant aspects of food intake as recommended by the National heart, Lung and Blood Institute (NHLBI), a part of the US Department of Health and Human Services, in its Special Newsweek publication called *Heart Health,* By Beth Howard.

Basically, it recommended 5 Foods to Eat More of . . .

To quote, "In general, nutritionists recommend the Mediterranean-type diet featuring fish, grains, fruits, vegetables, beans nuts and seeds. If your diet is different, consider adding these artery-clearing super foods to your table.

"'Fish. The American Heart Association recommends eating fish, particularly fatty fish like Salmon, mackerel, Albacore Tuna, at least twice a week. It's high on Omega 3 fatty acids, which may reduce the risk ofhem1 disease.

"'Soy. A recent meta-analysis from researchers at the Chinese university in Hongkong concluded that soy foods—such as soy nuts, soy milk, edamen and tempeh, may reduce total LOL (bad) cholesterol levels, while raising the (good) HOL cholesterol. The FDA allows soy food manufacturers to station their packaging that 25 grams of protein a day may reduce heart disease risks.

"Beans and Nuts. A new Harvard School of Public Health study found that one third of a cup of dried beans a day was associated with 38% percent for a second heart attack among a group of heart attack survivors.

Almonds, pecans and peanuts are all high in monosaturated fats, which help protect the heart. But limit your intake to handful (about 1.5 ounces a day).

"Oats. The fiber in oats both reduces the total LDL cholesterol levels and lower blood pressure—two heart disease risk factors.

"Garlic. This flavorful herb contains compounds that may help lower cholesterol levels. Research also suggests that garlic has some blood-thinning properties and anti-oxidant effects that may inhibit heart disease.

•••••••AND 3 TO SCRATCH

Minimize consumption of

"Red meat. It's one of the richest sources of artery-clogging saturated fats.

"Soda. Loaded with simple sugars and calories, sodas contribute to obesity among children and adults.

"French Fries. They contain both saturated and transfats. Says Dr. De Vane,·' They are making us fat and putting us at risk for heart attacks."

"Coffee & Cola: Good News/Bad News. Enjoy your java, ladies. It seems that the caffeine in coffee does not increase women's risk of hypertension. according to a study in *The Journal of the American Medical Association.* Using data from the Nurses' health School, it found no association between habitual coffee drinkers and the risk of developing high blood pressure. Dr. Winkelmeyer speculates that the many antioxidants known to be in coffee might offset the long-tenn detrimental effects of caffeine. The study did, however, found a link between hypertension and colas, both sugar-free and regular. The researchers suggest some compound in sodas other than caffeine responsible."

MY TAKE ON THESE SUGGESTIONS

In my earlier observations, I commented on the eating habits of Orientals and Occidentals—that is, Asians and North Americans. Southeast Asians, being surrounded by water and much arable land, have developed the habits of eating marine foods. cereals and vegetables. Rice and fish are basic staple foods. Milk and red meat are in scarce supply, hence not generally included in the people's diet. Many of course, drink tea or coffee. Older citizens were not addicted to colas. Obesity does not seem to be a general trait among them. On the other hand, western civilization have developed certain habits, basically consisting of more fatty intakes like fast-f-d and soda . . ., milk and red meats. Apparently, this translates into a higher percentage of a more obese population hence, the higher incidence of cholesterol-related ailments.

It may also be considered that certain exercise regimen in the Far East consisting of Aerobics and Bio-energy programs help to contribute for longer life and lower incidence of obesity-related diseases.

For our purpose, I have cited the foregoing health habits as a possible companion piece to our Suggested Light Aerobics and Breathing Dynamics for Seniors and the Lazy Man! In the later stages of our lives, it may not be immediately possible to reverse the ravages wrought by the abusive styles during our younger days but certainly, we could help arrest the damages to our well-being by taking advantage of the many discoveries in science and medicine. Perfecting and practicing our suggested Breathing Techniques for example, could help restore the efficacy of our body repair mechanisms and permit our vital organs to perform their assigned functions with better efficiency. This can be better achieved by the judicious usage of fresh oxygen to help replenish the fuel needs of the cells in our bloodstream. I noted that some practitioners of Tai Ichi would call this technique *Abdominal Breathing*.

My system simplifies this method into three easy steps, namely:

1. INHALE (INH)—slow suction of air into you system for 12 seconds.

2. HOLD DOWN AND PRESS (HDP)—Collect inhaled air at bottom of lungs Press and Hold it down for the next 30 Seconds.

3. EXHALE (EXH)—gradually exhale through the nose for 16 Seconds. or known as the *Arcebuche Breathing Cycle of 12-30-16.*

Chapter XVI

ARCEBUCHE—STYLE OF REGENERATIVE BREATHING CYCLES

How the *Arcebuche—Style* of Breathing Cycle can affect you.

Throughout this regimen, I have emphasized the need for my Breathing Techniques to be integrated as a necessary segment of this Light Aerobics exercise. Perhaps, readers will be able to better appreciate the system if I can share with them, the way in which it had a possible effects on me. I believe that in due time, and having mastered the *System* as recommended, it will eventually achieve the same advantages upon those who will practice this regimen. In my case, developing and mastering the techniques did not come overnight but a period of years of research, experimentation and practice. In fact, it was just in the last year that I have managed to organize and arrange the *system,* resulting in a more equitable physiological response, a feeling of healthier well-being and a more positive mental attitude did I felt confident enough to recommend it by writing this book.

a. Start off your Breathing Exercise with the 10-25-12 Breathing Cycle to done THREE (3) TIMES, interspaced with normal breathing BREAKS of three regular breathing Rate, before moving on to next Breathing Cycle: ergo: INHALE (IN) - 10 Seconds

HOLD AIR DOWN & PRESS (HDP) - 25 Seconds
EXHALE (EX) - 12 Seconds

Then, PAUSE for three (3) Regular Breathes & Proceed to next Breathing Cycle of 10-25-12.

b. This cycle is also your BASIC EXERCISE REGIMEN (10-25-12) such that during HDP, you should perform your Stretching Exercises, etc.. If 25 seconds is not enough, you may allow yourself to INHALE for another 5 seconds or more as needed, but DO NOT EXHALE until done with your stretching exercise.

c. For INTERMEDIATE EXERCISE REGIMEN, the Breathing Cycle should be 12-30-14. Warm-up Breathing Exercise should be performed FIVE (5) times -also interspaced with regular Breating Breaks if needed.

d. For ADVANCE EXERCISE REGIMEN, Breathing is 12-30-16. to be performed SEVEN (7) Times with Breathing breaks.

Chapter XVII

FAST FORWARD TO 2011

It was a balmy day of the last week of May, 2011, inside the Consultation clinic of my primary Cardiologist, Dr. Chris Y. Kim, MD, FACC at the seventh floor of Pikes Peak Cardiology Center at the sprawling Memorial Hospital in Colorado Springs. I was seated near the corner of the room facing the door. Ranged around me were my son, Vincent, his wife Brenna Allison Powers and good neighbor and perennial houseguest, Brenda Dorey. They were all in rapt attention as Dr.Kim outlined their findings about my heart condition. Earlier in the week, I was subjected to an Angioplasty operation to help determine, once and for all, of the real condition of my heart.

At my instance, a second opinion from his early diagnosis about arterial blockages, was confirmed by Dr. Chris Wehr, a cardiothoracic surgeon with lineages from Austria. He confirmed that two of my arteries were totally blocked (by plaque), while a third was 80% obstructed.

Trying to sound casual but professional, Dr. Kim outlined the potential dangers of delaying a heart by-pass operation. I told him earlier of my desire to first go home to the Philippines to see my ailing mother, relatives and other friends, after which, upon my return, I will submit to their suggestion.

My rationale is that, come what may, I have lived a full life. My initial budget (for life expectancy) was only up to age 60 (Being aware of my wilder years while young). After that time, it will be bonus years. I just needed to get home after a decade of absence from family and friends.

I reiterated my plan to them, with the hope that my request, being reasonable, will be granted. Vincent, Brenna and Brenda looked askance at the doctor. Dr. Kim. being of Korean descent, understood my desire to go home. However, when pressed about its advisability, he shrugged his shoulders and said "I can't make any guarantees to you. He could suffer a fatal attack any time and while over there in the Philippines, we can't do anything much for him! In fact, what I found surprising is that he lasted for over a decade until now, without having a heart attack or a deadly stroke. This is in fact, a very rare occurrence!"

I proudly explained to them, of my Light Aerobics Exercises of Deep Breathing and Stretching regimen which kept me feeling fit.

My son shook his head. "Dad, I havn't seen you perform any form of activity that can be described as a worthwhile exercise. In fact, you take too much coffee, eat unhealthy foods like pork, and spend much time in bed reading! You're reaping the fruits of years of inactivity, despite our incessant reminders!"

This brought a knowing smile from Dr.Kim.

A QUADRUPLE HEART BY-PASS OPERATION.

Vincent, asked for a few day's time to consult with his other siblings, and we headed for home.

After a series of conference calls with his elder brother, Michael of Cape Cod, MA, her elder sister Arlene C. Alvaran in Hyannis, MA and eldest sister, Lalaine C. Tamundong in Los Angeles, CA, they were unanimous in their collective decision to put me under the knife, prior to any trips scheduled for home.(He couldn't reach her other sister, Christina Arcebuche and her daughter, Lindsey). Drake Caballa Arcebuche, teenage son of the late James Nicholas Arcebuche and Inday Caballa, was also not contacted in Toronto, Ontario

The logic was it was a bit risky for me to traipse to far away Philippines, such that if I suffer an (heart) attack, they will be helpless to assist me.

Between my children and the Cardiological specialists, I had to give in. "Que Sera, Sera" I said. "Okay, if it will make you happy." And placed myself in the hands of the Lord! I think they were more nervous than me.

So, it came to pass that on June 1, 2011, exactly seventy years and five months to the day of my life, I went under the knife. Their earlier assessment for three blocked arteries, turned out to be incorrect, when upon opening me up, Dr. Chris Weir discovered a fourth suspicious artery—hence, his decision for a quadruple by-pass surgery. My son Vincent, his wife Brenna, neighbor Brenda and other friends came to visit and cheer me up in succeeding days. They echoed the doctor's comment that I now 'have a new heart!'. After a ten-day stay, I was released with the assurance that I will be getting regular visits from a homecare nurse and a Physical Therapist. My recovery was going fine, save for regular dizzy spells and incessant coughing. My cabinet was filled with numerous bottles of medicines I had to take daily. Medication failed to cure my dizziness. When I called my sister, Dolores (Baby) de la Cruz (who was herself having heart problems in the Philippines), she advised me to eat chicken or pork livers, gizzard and heart portions, interspersed with the egg whites (only) of hard-boiled eggs. I followed her suggestions and to my surprise, my dizzy spells abated.

(This advice, I included as # 16, on the Chapter—(Other Suggested Health Practices).

It may be useful at this time, to also point out that part of my fast recovery was in continuing on with my own Light Aerobics Exercise regimen—that of deep breathing and stretching activities. My home care nurse, Kristina Sharp was fascinated by the alternative modes I practiced that helped sped up my recovery. She claimed that I was a unique one from among her other patients. I simply grinned and told her about my system of Light Aerobics for Seniors and the Lazy Man!.

Chapter XIX

CONCLUDING SEGMENT

It will be safe at this stage, to introduce the *third* important component of this *system*. I found it appropriate enough to help celebrate the gift of intelligence and reason which is exclusive to man and denied to other living forms in this planet. Humans, unlike animals or plants, have a superior and more sophisticated degree of life. Where animals and insects survive on pure instincts, man goes a bit further by being able to think with logic, react to emotion, behave with reason and devise ways and means to help improve life even to incorporate ease, convenience, comfort and pleasure in them. Thus, our physical well-being is not only governed by the availability of food and proper environment, but is more complicated by our mental, emotional and psychological factors. Our entire system is governed by a more complex coordination of these interlocking influences, which in turn compels our body to behave or react accordingly.

For example, various stimuli like pleasure, stress, environment, personal relationships and a number of many other confliction emotions could cause the hypothalamus, the body's thermostat, to send appropriate signals to our various organs. These prompts, relayed through our nervous system, will trigger various reactions to increase, retard, stabilize, suppress chemical elements and processes which in turn help govern the motor functions of the entire coordinate systems. Consider *the fight or flight syndrome!*

Animals and insects for example, are not overtly affected by promotions, transfers or demotions at work, by fiscal bankruptcy or winning prizes in contests. When food or water are scare, they just moved on to find better sources, oftentimes by herd instincts. Dh, they do at times fight and compete for it, even the ritual of mating and herd superiority levels in seeming justification to the Darwinian theory for the survival of the fittest—but when push comes to shove, they just tend to accept their fate, to flee or lie down and die.

Daily life for the modern man or woman, gets increasingly competitive and complex. You have to learn to read and write, memorize words and phrases, to communicate in a babel of languages, learn to operate machinery, seek employment to supply yourself with food, habitations, clothes, communications, entertainment and mobility options; learn government laws. know more about your health and body, garbage and conservation, banking and finance, sports,—ad infinitum, ad nauseam! Could animals be better off? Not necessarily.

As I grew older (and hopefully, more matured), I have learned to appreciate the new pleasures in letting go—the capacity to be less attached to things, habits, relationships and possessions. When life deals me a bum card, I just call to mind the Serenity Poem"' Lord, grant me the Serenity to Accept the Things I cannot Change, the Courage to Change the Things I can and the Wisdom to Know the Difference! Most of our disappointments are basted on unrealized expectations. especially when we aim to set higher goals for ourselves then, fail to achieve them. We get excited and stressed, causing harm to our systems. Now, do you get the drift on how this relates to exercise?

The good news is that we can still take back control of our bodily functions at will. Consider this. More than two thousand years ago, the biblical injunction of Loving Thy neighbor as You love Thyself', was one simple and encompassing tenet for human relations ad advocated by Jesus Christ. This was echoed by Mohammad and many other prophets. Man however, is never content and developed vices—particularly the Seven Deadly Sins mentioned in Proverbs 6:16-19 consisting of Pride, Envy, Gluttony, Lust, Anger, Greed & Sloth! Most ofour grief can be traced to one or a combination of them.

When we pamper ourselves with these negative-inducing traits, we can be disappointed a primordial cause for system's dysfunction and ailment. It was true more than 2000 years ago and most certainly applicable and true today! Try slowly counting to 10, should you be tempted by the terrible Seven. They are not easy to deny.

One of the suggestions mentioned in the Other Suggested health Practices is "to think happy thoughts, avoid negative deeds or depressing situations, Get a grip on the Big Picture of Life," and Accent the Positive. You're not in the streets, in the hospital or in jail! The ancient medical sages, Galen and Solon proposed for physicians to "Heal thyself" This was no idle suggestion. The Oriental-style of meditations help to induce self-healing. Part of it is to remove distressing thoughts or situations. The system we propose works better when negative influences are replaced with happy and positive thoughts. Freemasonry, for example, emphasizes to its initiates, the observation of the Seven Cardinal Virtues as represented by Fortitude, Temperance, Prudence and Justice.

These are reinforced by the three tenets of Brotherly Love, Relief and Truth! The sincere concern of a mason for the welfare of his brethren is even extended to their widows and orphans! He is encouraged to be upright and moral in his ways, to "'meet on the leve; and part on the Square". This is reinforced by his unbridled love for liberty and equality and his trusting relationship with his Creator. These are all the basis upon which the superstructure of Freemasonry is erected and anchored upon. This runs counter to the Seven Cardinal Sins that project negative vibes, causing grief all around. Masonic virtues are being cited for the positive virtues it inculcates for a more pleasant relationship with family and neighbors. This also help us to take better control of our lives. We all know these, but the lure to the destructive adherence of vices and superfluities in life compels us to embrace the momentary pleasures with the Seven Deadly Sins as against the lasting joy in "loving they neighbor as you love yourself"

These reminders are not included her for moralizing purposes. This is not our objective. There are priests, ministers, imams, grandparents and well-meaning neighbors who can better influence our behavior. Rather, we are attempting to set the grou7ndwork for the ideal conditions in which our *System* can thrive and made effectively put to work for your own benefit. If you love your body enough, there should be no half-measures in the way you should treat it. When you love a toy or a car, you do not abuse or neglect them. You can do no less for your body.

Readers are further encouraged to know their bodies more intimately—to reintroduce and reacquaint themselves with their bodies. Remember the familiar refrain "I've been to Paradise, but I've never been to me"? Why is it paradoxical for some people to marginalize or neglect those they love? Can we not be better and be above this petty weakness? I used to tell my children "your reason is good, but the result is not!" There are some ways in knowing yourself. Now, let's go to work.

1. Read books and literatures about the human body (See Recommended Readings References). These are informative topics in the Internet and even entertaining programs on television like the National Geographic, Discovery, Science and History Channels. Remember that "Information is knowledge and Knowledge is Power."

2. Know what's ailing you and learn more about it. This precious commodity, your body, must not be entrusted solely to the responsibility of outside opinions. Your physicians can only be as effective as the kind and completeness of the information you provide them about yourself. Learning more about the way your system works can make you better understand and appreciate how to alleviate your ailments. Forearmed, you can even "will" or induce the ailing organs to regenerate themselves through our exercise regimen by helping feed your cells with oxygen-laden air through our Breathing Dynamics, which facilitates the absorption of nutrients and ejecting wastes. Positive and happy thoughts enable the brain to send effective messages for the production of repair and regenerative enzymes or chemicals.

3. One untapped source are brochures and literatures accompanying prescription medicines or drug packets for certain ailments.

You can also read on them as advertised in newspapers and magazines. It provides specific advices about the functions of the various elements comprising the drug, its medicinal roles and caveats. These are reliable findings culled through experiments and tests approved by the FDA. We are in fact cautioned against the wanton introduction of foreign objects that can be harmful to the human body. Exercise and proper breathing as advocated in this regimen, is one natural way to perform the healing process. When we do something your body abhors, like the indeterminate use of alcohol, tobacco or drugs; an abusive lifestyle or diet, we are duly informed. Its warning systems are manifested by colds, headaches, pains, itchiness, chills, blemishes, lesions, tiredness, muscular weakness, etc. When ignored or left untreated, it progresses to more serious forms of ailments. When you commit a crime, there are times you can get away with it however, authorities or society will eventually catch up with you. Still, you have the privilege of prior knowledge. It is called "conscience".

4. In both cases involving social interaction and those relating to your body, being aware of what you are about to do gives you the element or opportunity of control, thus being affording the following options:

    a.) Prevent it

    b.) Apply palliative measures

    c.) If damage has already been done, take remedial steps.

    d.) When made aware, do not permit the damage to run its course, to continue and deteriorate, as repairs can be harder and costly down the line. Seek the advice of others—of specialists, authorities rather than perform self-medication or DIY (Do It yourself). e) If you desire to cure yourself, do it from a position of strength by being smart enough to know its causes and effects.

Our suggested regimen of Light Aerobics and Breathing Dynamics calls for a parallel effort on your part to be consciously aware of what you are about to do. This means the proper ambiance or atmosphere for our system to function effectively. It is not like a magic pill you can swallow. In this setting, your bio-energy, the belief in the superiority of your "will" and your determination to take back control, will do the rest. Working in tandem with your physicians is also advised as you will be better off on the same wavelength. Even the best doctors and medications can only do so much. In the end, most will really still be u p to you. Once you learn more about your body, you can better harness your exercise regimen and "project" the curative strength of your "will" upon yourself, and even to others nearby or from a distance. In due time, you can become more confident, assertive and powerful.

How you react and benefit from this program will largely depend upon the level of practice and proficiency you manage to attain. As earlier explained, more than anyone else, you are best source of information on how it responds to your ministrations. When feeling relaxed and buoyant after a Breathing or Cooling-down session, then your body is now responding to the benefits of raised oxygen levels in your system. With judicious health habits, you can be a healthier and more fulfilled individual. To reiterate an earlier observation, you and I have but One Chance for life in this world. The quality on how we spend the rest of our final years will ultimately depend upon how we nurture and nourish the very system that make it all possible—our human body! Let's take back control. Let's breathe, exercise, live the proper lifestyles, to be healthy and happy for the rest of our days!

RECOMMENDED READING REFERENCES

Aerobics: **Aerobics Program For Total Well-Being: Exercise, Diet and Emotional Balance**

By Dr. Kenneth H. Cooper, MD, MPH (Bantam Books) also M.Evans & Co.,Inc. New York

Bio-Energy & Self-Healing: (Tetada) **KALIMASADA International: HQ** Surabaya, Indonesia

Grand Master PAK EDDY SUROHADI & Master Dr. Ida Widyastuti Surohadi
Also Check with **YOU TUBE** on **KALIMASDA** for Video & other Details.

Breathing: **Go to Website on Deep Breathing**

"Light Aerobics Exercises for Seniors and the Lazy Man!"—*Arcebuche Breathing Style*

D I e t : **Three-Day Nutritional Facelift**—By Dr. Nicholas NV Perricone

Center For Food Safety & Applied Nutrition—By The US Food & Drug Administration

Exercise : **The No-Sweat Exercise Plan**—By: Dr. Harvey Simon

Pranic Healing : **The Ancient Sciences and Art of Pranic Healing**— By Masster Choa Kok Sui

The Human Anatomy, Wellness and Health: **Wellness—Concepts & Health (Second Edition)** By: David Anspaugh, Michael Hamrick & FrankRosato.

The Doctor's Book of Food Remedies. Also Doctors 100 All-Time Greatest Home

Remedies—(Available through **Prevention** Magazine of Harlan, IA 51593-3740.)

The Pillbook, the Illustrated guide to . . . . 11ᵗʰ, 12ᵗʰ & future editions— By CMD Publishing/ Bantam Dell (Random House)

The Truth About Six-Pack Abs—By Mike Geary *help-desk@truthaboutabs.com*

Healthwise Handbook (A self-Care Handbook For You) By: Humana Military Healthcare Services/ TRICARE Heartland—By Donald W.Kemper. MPH

Health For Life (Newsweek) & HeartHealth (*www.nhlbi.nih.gov*)

Illustrated Book Of The Human Anatomy—For Nursing & Medical Students)

Spiritual Upliftment:

The Power of Intention; Getting In The Gap (& other books) By Dr. Wayne W. Dyer

Chapter XX

READERS' OPTIONAL INPOUTS FOR EVALUATION;

NAME: _____ A G E (Optional) _____
ADDRESS: _____
_____

Email: _____ Tel Nos. _____

Q U E S T I O N N A I R E:

1. Do you perform any type of exercise program at this time?
    _____
    (If so, what type and how often?)
    _____

2. Are You presently taking any form of prescribed medications, vitamins, supplements or other non-prescribed alternative medication (How often) for any type of ailment?
    (If so, please list in a separate sheet and attached it to this questionnaire)

3. In your voluntary acceptance and practice of the exercise regimen or any portion thereof, what kind of ailment (s) do you expected to be alleviated from?

    Ailment Type   Since When?   Severity Level (Scale of 1-10)
    _____   _____   _____
    _____   _____   _____
    _____   _____   _____

    (Note : Use separate sheet if you have additional comments about the above)

I confirm that all the answers to the above questions are true to the best of my ability and hold the author or his representatives blameless and free from any form of damages, torts, suits or complaints of any kind for any form of harm or injury to my person or anyone else not under their direct supervision.

(Signature)_____ Date: _____

ABOUT THE AUTHOR: JAIME ESTREMERA ARCEBUCHE

For much of his life, the author was involved in machinery and engineering works. He took courses in Farm Mechanics at the University of Eastern Philippines and Mechanical Engineering at the FEATI University. He worked with the U. S. Industries (Philippines), Inc., the local dealer for Caterpillar, John Deere, Mack Trucks and other allied equipment after finishing a company-sponsored four-year Apprenticeship Training Program. He had stints in the Service, Parts Sales and Promotion Departments, his last assignment as a Field Service Training Instructor for outside customers and in-house trainees. Later, he established his own company specializing in the sales and servicing of turbochargers. He also spent two decades developing a fuel-saver device. His prototype helped increase his vehicle mileage by 33%, lower exhaust emission particulates by 40% raised acceleration by 15% and was granted a Probational Patent by the U. S. Patent Office. Meanwhile, he found time for civic and fraternal groups, appointed a District Deputy Grandmaster, presiding officer of the Scottish Rite (33rd) and York rite concordant bodies as well as an active member of the Shrine (AAONMS).

In the last decade, much of his time was devoted to the study of wellness and health, researching on various books and publications about Oriental and Western authors about the subject. He was one of the Maharishi Yogi Select Group of 7000 practitioners, an accredited member of the Philippines Institute of Traditional and Alternative Health Practices and completed the basic course in Indonesian exercise regimen of Tetada Kalimasada—an ancient method of inner energy cultivation and self-induced therapy. For a time, he gave exercise instructions to Senior Citizens in Tennessee and Kentucky. He has six children and ten grandchildren. The author now lives in Fountain City, Colorado.